Heart Disease

What it is and How it's Treated

John Wallwork and Rob Stepney

Heart Disease

What it is and How it's Treated

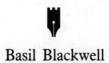

Basil Blackwell

Copyright © John Wallwork and Rob Stepney 1987

First published 1987

Basil Blackwell Ltd
108 Cowley Road, Oxford, OX4 1JF, UK

Basil Blackwell Inc.
432 Park Avenue South, Suite 1503
New York, NY 10016, USA

British Library Cataloguing in Publication Data

Wallwork, John
  Heart disease : what it is and how it's
  treated.
  1. Heart—Diseases
  I. Title   II. Stepney, Rob
  616.1′2   RC681

  ISBN 0–631–14884–1
  ISBN 0–631–14885–X Pbk

Library of Congress Cataloging in Publication Data

Wallwork, John, 1946–
  Heart disease : what it is and how it's treated.

  Includes index.
  1. Heart—Diseases—Popular works. 2. Cardiology—
Popular works. I. Stepney, Rob. II. Title.
[DNLM: 1. Cardiology—popular works. WG 113 W215h]
RC681.W3 1986   616.1′2   86–17645
ISBN 0–631–14884–1
ISBN 0–631–14885–X (pbk.)

Typeset in 10 on 12pt Plantin
by Photo Graphics, Honiton, Devon
Printed in Great Britain

Contents

About the Authors

John Wallwork attended medical school in Scotland, and trained in heart surgery in Edinburgh and Glasgow. After that, he worked in Adelaide for six months and then for two years in Stanford, California, under Professor Norman Shumway, gaining experience in heart and heart–lung transplants. He returned to work in Britain in 1981, becoming Consultant Cardiothoracic Surgeon at Papworth Hospital, Cambridge.

Rob Stepney is a medical and science writer and journalist. He was special correspondent for *World Medicine*, and has contributed articles to the *Sunday Times, Guardian, New Scientist, New Society* and the BBC. He edits *Murmurs*, a cardiology newsletter, and is contributing editor of *Pharmacy Update*. He was educated at Oxford, Newcastle and Cambridge universities.

Acknowledgements

We are very grateful to cardiologists Dr Ian Brooksby, of the Norfolk and Norwich Hospital, and Dr Ross Lorimer, of Glasgow Royal Infirmary, who read an earlier manuscript of this book and offered useful amendments and comment. Ben Milstein, emeritus consultant cardiothoracic surgeon at Papworth Hospital, also contributed valuable ideas. We thank Dr David Zideman (from the Hammersmith Hospital) and the Resuscitation Council for allowing us to publish their brochure as an appendix.

Introduction

If you are reading this book because you have heart disease, or because a friend or relative is affected by it, you will find advice on how to cope with the problem and how to aid recovery. If you do not have heart disease, we hope that there is information and understanding here to help prevent it.

Though not much larger than a clenched fist, the heart's daily 100,000 beats circulate almost 2,000 gallons of blood. In a year, this extraordinary pump beats non-stop between 30 and 40 million times – in a lifetime, two and a half billion times. In its tirelessness and reliability, the heart is an example of supreme biological engineering. But, as with any engine, it relies on its components. The heart has chambers that collect and distribute blood, valves that regulate its flow, muscle that provides power, an electrical system to control the timing of the whole process and piping that supplies the heart muscle itself with blood, and so with the oxygen and nutrients it needs for fuel.

Any or all of these components may fail: chambers may have holes, valves may leak, muscle may become flabby and electrical circuits are liable to disconnections and short-circuits. Each problem gives rise to a different form of heart disease. But the most common difficulty is with the heart's own fuel supply. It arises because the vessels serving the heart muscle – the coronary arteries – become lined with fatty deposits which restrict and ultimately block the flow of blood. Without sufficient blood, there is too little oxygen and food for the heart tissues. It is this that leads to the pain of angina, and the death of heart muscle in a heart attack (or 'coronary') that can fatally cripple the heart's ability to function. Around eight out of ten patients with cardiac problems have disease of the heart's coronary arteries.

Fortunately, as we have come to understand more about the heart, we have been able to develop ways of intervening to aid its work, and repair or replace its component parts. This has revolutionised the outlook in almost every aspect of heart disease.

Over 120 drugs are available to influence the way the heart and circulatory system function: many reduce the effect of coronary disease by expanding the heart's blood vessels or by reducing its need for oxygen. Artificial electrical devices regulate the rate at which the heart beats; plastic, metal or animal valves replace those that are stiff or leaking; and blood vessels taken from other parts of the body are used to restore the heart's own blood supply. Most dramatically of all, within the past two years – and after a decade of critical evaluation – we have become able to offer heart transplantation as a routine clinical service in certain kinds of heart failure where no other therapy can help.

Impressive though the achievements of medicine and surgery have been, dealing with heart disease often involves difficult choices. After one heart attack, is it worth taking drugs – perhaps for many years – in an attempt to prevent another? When is the best time to replace a damaged heart valve? Will surgery for the chest pain of angina afford a greater chance of long life? This book aims to provide information to help patients understand their doctor's advice when it comes to making such decisions. It is also written in the belief that our knowledge, attitudes and behaviour affect our chances of developing heart disease and influence what will happen if we do.

The form and function of the healthy heart are explained in chapter 1, and the general kinds of problem that can arise in chapter 2. What the heart does in health and illness is so closely linked to the way it is constructed that one cannot be understood without the other. Chapter 1 is essential reading; so are parts of chapter 2 (though the sections dealing specifically with heart defects present at birth and with infectious diseases of the heart will be relevant only to a minority). Chapter 3, on methods of diagnosis, is also important. Doctors use a range of tests and investigations to establish exactly what has gone wrong and what can best be done about it. Some of these techniques may be intimidating until their nature and purpose are explained.

The book then considers particular types of heart problem, beginning with heart attacks and angina. These conditions are two facets of the same disease: blockage of the coronary arteries causing the heart muscle to be starved of blood. We then examine abnormalities of heart rate and rhythm, which will be of particular interest to anyone who needs or already has a pacemaker. This is followed by a chapter on heart valves in which the need for surgery and the advantages and disadvantages of different types of valve replacement are discussed. There is then an account of measures that can be taken to help the failing heart and of heart transplants. Chapter 11 provides a glimpse of new methods of treatment which may become widespread over the next decade.

Most of our heart problems arise from disease of the coronary arteries. Yet in our grandparents' time coronary artery disease was rare – and still is in many countries. This is evidence that its origins lie (at least partly) in our style of life. Certain behaviours – particularly smoking – are clearly preventable, self-inflicted risks. However, the role of other factors, and the importance of diet in particular, are still controversial. Chapter 12 presents both sides of the argument about heart disease prevention.

High blood pressure increases the risk of heart disease and so is also considered in chapter 12. Drugs used to treat this common condition are described in the last chapter. High blood pressure may affect many different organs in the body; in this book we deal with it only as it relates to heart disease.

The final chapter gives a thorough account of the confusing range of medicines available to treat heart disease, and the book ends with appendices which describe what happens during open-heart surgery, the rules relating to driving with a heart condition, and how to help someone who has collapsed with heart disease. The addresses of organisations that work to prevent heart disease and help those who suffer from it are given.

Unless otherwise specified, figures given to describe the heart and its work – the amount of blood it pumps, for example – relate to a middle-aged man of average height and weight. The heart's size and workload are usually smaller in women.

Chapter One

The Healthy Heart

In our imagination, the heart swells with love, breaks in misery, is strong in those who are brave, warm in the friendly and cold in the unfeeling. In reality, it is simply an efficient, compact, tireless and extremely reliable pump: fluid flows in at one end and is expelled at the other. But perhaps because at times of greatest emotion we can actually feel the heart move, it seems to embody what is unique about life itself, and has come to symbolise so much of human experience.

The liver and kidneys are just as essential to our survival, yet seem far less important. The extent of this difference in attitude is clear from our response to major heart operations. While kidney and liver surgery goes largely unnoticed, operations on the heart have long been headline news. For many years we thought of life as ending when the heart stopped – even though, as we now accept, it is when the brain ceases to function that a person is truly dead. Perhaps these special feelings for the heart are legacies of the time when it was considered the seat of the soul or of our conscience. In a pharoah's tomb, for example, a wall painting shows the dead king's heart being weighed on a pair of scales to determine whether the balance of good or evil would admit him to heaven.

Our knowledge of what the heart actually does is relatively recent. The Greek philosopher Aristotle thought that the flame of life, which provided the warmth so characteristic of the living body and so absent in the dead, literally burned within its chambers. For Galen, a Roman doctor, the heart was like a blast furnace, turning physical food into the spiritual substance which actually 'worked' the body. The lungs were thought of as bellows, aiding the smelting process.

It was not until William Harvey's discovery of the circulation of the blood in the early seventeenth century that the heart's true nature – that of a pump – became clear. It was later still that the role of the lungs was appreciated. Just as a candle flame requires oxygen to burn, so the cells of the body need oxygen to provide the energy they use to live and work. And, just as a flame would be stifled by the build up of carbon dioxide, the body's cells would be poisoned if the waste products of combustion were not removed. Blood must therefore be circulated not only to the body but also to the lungs, where the gases it carries can be exchanged with those in the air, before it is once again pumped around the body.

The two pumps

The heart is often thought of as a single pump. But since there are two circulations – one to the lungs and one to the body – the heart is in fact two pumps, lying side by side. Blood flows from the body into the heart, and is propelled from there into the lungs. It returns to the heart's second pump and is then circulated to the body. This simple cycle of events is shown in figure 1.1.

So that blood does not build up on one side of the heart or the other, the two pumps have the same capacity – around 70 cc, which is roughly equivalent to the volume of a wine glass. The amount pumped with each heart beat is not large relative to the total volume of blood (around 4 litres, or 8 pints) in our bodies. Frequent beating

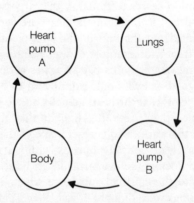

Figure 1.1 The heart consists of two pumps, shown here as A and B.

is therefore vital if the circulation is to be maintained. The two heart pumps are similar in construction. Both consist of two chambers: an atrium, which collects blood flowing into the heart, and a main pumping chamber, the ventricle, which pumps it out again. Figures 1.2 and 1.3 map the circulation in more detail and begin to show the basic structure of the heart. Incidentally, doctors label the heart from the patient's point of view, and not from that of someone looking at him. So the right side is the side that is on *your* right, as you 'look out' from your body. This means that diagrams of the heart, which is always portrayed from the front, show the right atrium and ventricle on the left of the page.

The pump on the right feeds blood to the lungs through the pulmonary artery. This blood then returns to the heart rich in oxygen. The pump on the left sends oxygenated blood into a large artery called the aorta. From there, smaller arteries branch off, taking the blood coursing through the rest of the body. In the body's tissues, the oxygen and nutrients carried by the fresh blood are exchanged for carbon dioxide and chemical waste. Blood carrying these substances returns through the network of veins to the right side of the heart. Carbon dioxide is then exchanged for oxygen in the lungs, and waste products are filtered out by the kidneys as the blood makes its next circuit of the body. Blood cells accomplish a single circuit of body and lungs in less than 60 seconds.

One-way flow

A system of valves ensures that blood circulates in the required direction (*see* figure 1.3). Once an atrium has filled, blood is passed into the ventricle through a valve, consisting of two or three thin but strong flaps of tissue shaped like the petals of a flower. As with any other flap valve, passage is in one direction only. When blood has filled the ventricle, the valves separating the pumping chamber from the atrium snap shut to ensure blood cannot return to the collecting chamber when the ventricle contracts.

The main work of the heart – pumping blood around the body – is the responsibility of the thick muscle walls of the left ventricle. From here, blood is ejected with the greatest force, and the heart valves are under most strain. Separating left atrium and left ventricle is the mitral valve, so called because its two flaps resemble a bishop's mitre. There is also a second vital valve which seals off the left

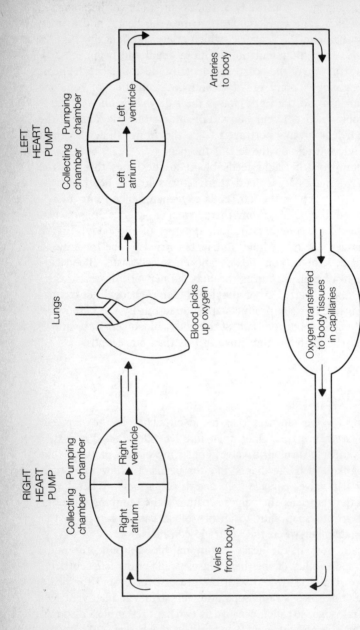

Figure 1.2 The right heart pumps blood to the lungs and the left heart serves the rest of the body. Both pumps are divided into two: a collecting chamber (atrium) into which blood flows, and a pumping chamber (ventricle) which expels it.

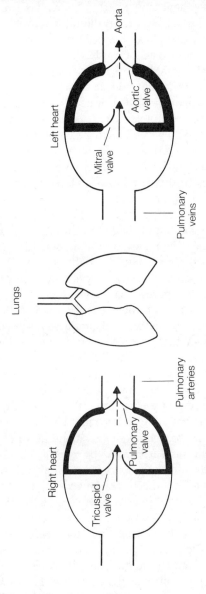

Figure 1.3 Acting like trap doors that can be pushed open only one way, four valves ensure that blood moves in only one direction through the heart. The valves open and shut in sequence, allowing blood to pass from the collecting chambers to the pumping chambers, and then from the pumping chambers out of the heart. Here, the tricuspid and mitral valves are open as blood flows from collecting to pumping chambers. Pulmonary and aortic valves are closed, preventing the return of blood pumped out by the previous beat.

ventricle once blood has been pumped into the aorta. If it were not for this aortic valve, blood would flow back into the heart when the left ventricle relaxed, without taking part in the circulation. Similar valves prevent blood flowing back from the right ventricle into the right atrium, and ensure that blood pumped from the right ventricle into the pulmonary arteries reaches the lungs.

We have considered the heart in simple terms as two pumps. These pumps are, of course, arranged side by side as a single organ. As it lies in the chest (figure 1.4), the heart is shaped like a blunt cone which has been tipped to one side. It is larger at the top and back where the atria are, and becomes narrower where the ventricles project slightly forwards and downwards. Surrounding the heart is a tough protective sac of tissue, called the pericardium, within which the heart moves freely. The heart is placed in the centre of the chest and is covered by the lungs.

Figure 1.4 shows the weaving 'figure of eight' path taken by blood as it passes into and out of the heart, through the lungs and back again. Its course can be followed in more detail in figure 1.5.

Blood returns from the body into the right atrium (1). Having given up its oxygen, blood at this stage appears burgundy red (but is usually coloured blue in figures). With a gentle squeeze, the right atrium contracts to push blood through the tricuspid (three-leaved) valve into the right ventricle (2). When the right ventricle contracts, blood is forced through the pulmonary artery to the lungs (3). (Vessels that carry blood away from the heart are always called arteries; those that carry blood to the heart are always veins.)

The lungs allow one gas (carbon dioxide) to be exchanged for another (oxygen). To do this efficiently, they must expose the maximum possible amount of blood to air. This is achieved by having increasingly fine, branching airways that end in clusters of tiny sacs, each of which is surrounded by minute blood vessels. This gives the healthy lung the appearance of a pink, air-filled sponge. When expanded to their greatest extent, the lungs can contain 5 litres of air, and the interface between air and blood has the same surface area as a tennis court.

From the lungs, blood flows back into the heart through the pulmonary veins (4). Rich with oxygen, it now appears bright red. Blood then passes through the mitral valve into the left ventricle (5), the main pumping chamber of the heart. As the left ventricle contracts, pressure of blood forces the mitral valve shut; the aortic valve opens, and blood surges into the aorta (6). Even when the

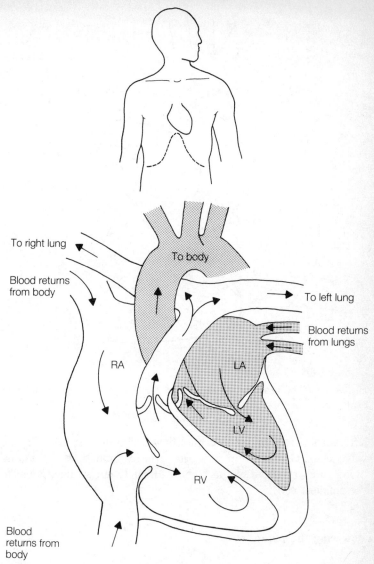

Figure 1.4 The heart's position in the chest and its structure. So that they fit into a compact space within the chest, the two pumps are arranged alongside each other and the blood vessels 'twisted' around them to make the necessary connections. RA = right atrium, RV = right ventricle, LA = left atrium, LV = left ventricle. The stippled area shows the presence of blood rich in oxygen.

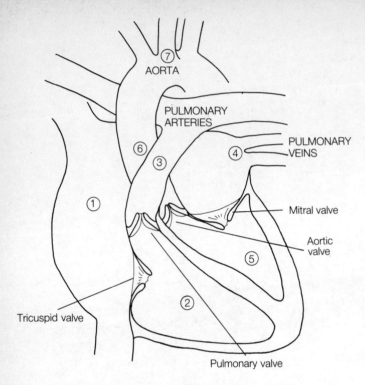

Figure 1.5 The heart valves and major blood vessels. The numbers are explained in the text.

left ventricle relaxes, blood cannot flow back into it since the aortic valve snaps closed. From the aorta, arteries branch off (7), taking blood to every organ of the body, ultimately supplying oxygen to the smallest cell.

Powering the pump

The walls of the heart are formed of a unique type of muscle. Each muscle fibre is capable of rhythmic contraction, and – on its own – each one will 'beat'. Placed together, the fibres' activity is synchronised, so that instead of working in an uncoordinated way they combine their resources, producing a contraction strong enough to send 8 pints or more of blood coursing around the body every minute. The period of contraction during which blood is expelled from the heart is called *systole* (pronounced 'systoly'), and the phase of relaxation that follows, *diastole* (pronounced 'diastoly').

Each heart cell works far harder than other muscle, and because of this has a great appetite for oxygen and nutrients. But the most remarkable feature of heart muscle is that its fibres – despite their rapidly repeated rhythmic contraction – do not tire. In this respect, the heart is quite unlike other muscle in the body. As with all muscle, the contraction of heart fibres is caused by an electrical impulse. A later section explains how the electrical current that drives the heart is generated and conducted.

Since the left ventricle has the most difficult job – that of powering blood at high pressure around the body – it is here that the heart muscle is most robust. At about 1 centimetre across, the wall of the left ventricle is three times as thick as that of the right ventricle.

Heart rate

Heart rate at rest changes with age. A child's heart beats relatively fast: around 100 times each minute at the age of three. In early adulthood the rate slows to about 70 beats (and far less than that in trained athletes); but it tends to increase again in the elderly. Both in these long-term changes, and over the short term, the healthy heart responds to the body's needs.

While resting or asleep, the organs of the body work at a reduced rate and require less food and oxygen. The heart therefore beats slowly. With moderate exercise or in times of excitement, heart rate may rise dramatically, and athletes are able to reach rates of 200 beats per minute for short periods. (A rough guide to an average person's maximum heart rate is 220 beats minus their age.) Heart rate, obvious to us as the pulse that we feel at the wrists, is the clearest evidence we have of the heart adjusting to changing demands. But it is not the only mechanism of self-regulation.

Moving blood around the body is like taking people up a mountain on a continuous ski-lift. Faced with more people wanting to use it, the operator can respond by making the lift go round faster, or keep it at the same speed but load more people onto each passing car. When the body demands more blood, the heart adjusts in both of these ways, increasing the rate at which it pumps, and also increasing the amount of blood pumped with each heart beat.

When we rest, our heart pumps a total of about 5 litres (roughly 1 gallon) of blood each minute. With exercise and anxiety, this rises three or four times, and athletes can achieve a cardiac output well in excess of 25 litres (or 5 gallons) per minute. (The output of the heart is calculated by measuring the amount of blood pumped with each beat and multiplying by the heart rate.)

A variety of mechanisms is involved in the control of cardiac output. One is the heart's ability to respond to the amount of blood arriving through the veins. Exercise results in more blood flowing back to the heart, which stretches the walls of the ventricles. The more heart muscle fibres are stretched (up to a certain point), the more powerfully they contract. This feedback mechanism therefore increases the volume of blood pumped out.

Other methods of control involve the nervous system. There are in fact two systems of nerves acting on the heart: one (called the *parasympathetic*) tends to slow heart rate, and the other (the *sympathetic*) to speed it up. Heart rate depends on the balance between the two. Under normal, resting conditions the net effect of nervous control is a slight braking action on the heart rate. But the mere sight of danger or excitement activates the sympathetic system and produces an immediate rise in heart rate.

There is also a system of chemical messengers (hormones) carried in the blood that conveys similar information, though more slowly than a direct nervous connection. The two hormones principally involved in increasing heart rate are adrenaline and noradrenaline (called epinephrine and norepinephrine in North America). These substances are the classic 'fight or flight' chemicals that prepare the body for exertion when danger threatens.

The way the heart is wired

In the laboratory, animal hearts that have been carefully removed continue to beat for days if provided with sufficient oxygen and nutrients. This is because the basic rhythm of the heart – the contraction and relaxation of atria and ventricles at appropriate points in the heart cycle – is inbuilt. Maintaining this rhythm is the job of specialised cells that are capable both of contracting (like muscle cells) and of conducting electricity (like nerves). Together, these cells form the electrical wiring system of the heart, regularly triggering contraction of the heart muscle by discharging small currents of electricity. (Each discharge is less than one-hundredth of a volt.) This 'wiring' system is shown in figure 1.6.

In normal rhythm, the order of events in the heart is precisely controlled so that the collecting chambers beat first, followed by the main pumping chambers. In this way the ventricles are 'topped up' with blood before they contract, and the heart works at maximum efficiency. It might be thought that the right side of the heart pumps blood first, followed by the left. But this is not the case. The two collecting chambers contract at much the same time, and then the two pumping chambers. So, as the right ventricle is contracting to send blood to the lungs, the left ventricle is contracting to send around the body blood that passed through the right ventricle a few seconds before.

Each beat begins in the heart's natural pacemaker, a collection of cells in the right atrium known as the *sinus node*. (Normal heart

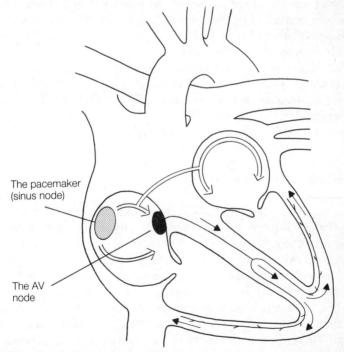

The pacemaker
(sinus node)

The AV
node

Figure 1.6 The 'wiring' of the heart. Arrows show the way the electrical impulse moves along the conduction pathways to the tip of the ventricles and then back along the muscle walls.

rhythm is therefore called sinus rhythm.) In the healthy heart, this pacemaker controls the rate of contraction: whatever rate it sets, the rest of the heart will follow. Ultimately, control of heart rate and rhythm lies with the electrical system of the heart. Changes that occur because of instructions from the nervous system and hormones must all be channelled through this mechanism.

The electrical impulse generated by the sinus node spreads relatively slowly (at 2–3 feet per second) through the two atria, bringing about a gentle contraction which fills the ventricles with blood. The electrical impulse is then delayed and concentrated in another collection of cells, known as the atrioventricular (or AV) node, which acts as a form of trigger. From there, dispersal of the current throughout both ventricles is by three specialised conduction pathways. Electricity moves along these fibres about five times faster than it spreads through the atria.

The purpose of the conduction fibres is to carry the electrical impulse quickly to the far end of the ventricles, so that muscle in this area contracts first. The wave of contraction then moves swiftly and powerfully upwards, squeezing blood out of the ventricles and into the large vessels that carry it away from the heart.

The entire passage of electric current through the heart can be recorded from the surface of the body, a recording known as an electrocardiogram (ECG or EKG). The events we have just described form the basis of the standard ECG pattern, shown in figure 1.7. More information about the ECG is given in chapter 3.

Bringing fuel to the heart

The heart is compact, flexible in the amount of work it can do and enormously reliable. But, like any pump, it does not work for free. The heart requires energy to fuel its own muscle, and it has to obtain its oxygen and nutrients by maintaining an adequate supply of blood. Though the heart is a small organ, it accounts for about 10 per cent of the body's consumption of oxygen.

The blood vessels that serve the heart muscle begin near the base of the aorta (figure 1.8) and follow shallow, fat-filled grooves on the heart surface that mark the boundaries between the heart chambers underneath. Smaller blood vessels branch off from the main channels, forming a dense network and penetrating the full thickness of the heart muscle beneath. These blood vessels are called coronary

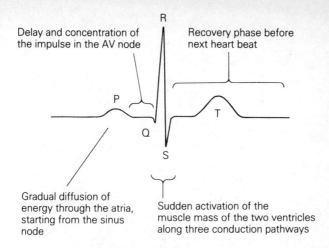

R

Delay and concentration of
the impulse in the AV node

Recovery phase before
next heart beat

P

T

Q

S

Gradual diffusion of
energy through the atria,
starting from the sinus
node

Sudden activation of the
muscle mass of the two ventricles
along three conduction pathways

Figure 1.7 The normal ECG. Each element in the waveform is assigned a letter. Because the ventricles represent a large mass of muscle, the 'complex' formed by the Q, R and S waves is large. The delay between contraction of the atria and contraction of the ventricles is about one-fifth of a second.

arteries since (like a crown) they start near the top of the heart and encircle it. Though only a few millimetres in diameter, the coronary arteries are among the most vital blood vessels in the body.

Initially there are two – right and left – though the left coronary artery divides so quickly that we usually think in terms of three major blood vessels. Figure 1.8 is a simplified view of the outside of the heart, showing where the coronary arteries begin and how they cover the front and back of the heart. Though the main coronary arteries are generally found in a similar place, there is great variation from one person to another in the way the smaller branches form.

Usually, all three major blood vessels take part in supplying blood to the heart's main beating chamber, the left ventricle. The blood vessel in figure 1.8 that runs the length of the heart (the left anterior descending artery) supplies a large amount of cardiac muscle at the front, and also the wall that divides the two beating chambers. It therefore plays a crucial role. The side walls of the heart are supplied by branches of the circumflex artery (that splits off from the left

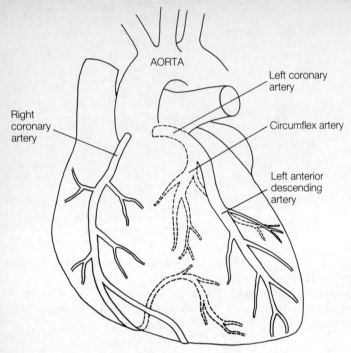

Figure 1.8 The main coronary arteries encircle the heart muscle, supplying it with blood-borne oxygen and nutrients.

coronary artery soon after it leaves the aorta); and the base of the left ventricle is usually served by the right coronary artery.

However, these arrangements differ from person to person. One of the most common variations (found in one in five people) is where the right coronary artery plays little or no part in supplying the left ventricle, which therefore relies on branches from the other two arteries alone. It is clear from these arrangements that blockages occurring in each blood vessel will have very different effects on the heart, and that the amount of damage done by coronary artery disease may vary considerably from one person to another.

Blood, arteries and veins

Ceaseless circulation of blood is needed to deliver oxygen and nutrients to the tissues, and to collect from them carbon dioxide and waste products. If there is no flow of blood to provide these two services, the organs of the body cannot survive.

Blood has two major constituents: cells and the fluid in which those cells are carried. Red cells – responsible for carrying oxygen in their haemoglobin, which is a red-coloured pigment – form the majority of the cell population. The remainder consists of white cells, of many different types, which defend us against infection and are involved in inflammation. There are also cellular components (rather than proper cells) that are essential to blood clotting and the initial stages of blood vessel repair. These components are called platelets. The fluid in which the blood cells circulate makes up about 60 per cent of blood volume. Known as plasma, it is this fluid that transports nutrients to (and waste products from) body tissues. It also contains important substances that influence blood clotting. Some of these special proteins exist to aid clotting when blood vessels are damaged; others are designed to prevent clotting in normal vessels. The two kinds of substance exist in a delicate balance.

When the left ventricle contracts, blood leaves the heart and enters the aorta, the body's largest artery. It is travelling at a speed of roughly 1 metre (3 feet) per second and is under considerable pressure. The first organ the heart supplies with fresh blood is itself. Close to the origin of the aorta are small openings in its wall marking the start of the coronary arteries (*see* figure 1.8).

Some 4 centimetres further on, at the top of the arch of the aorta, are three branches which themselves divide to feed blood to the brain (which takes about one-eighth of the heart's output), the head and the arms. The aorta then turns the corner and starts to descend through the trunk of the body, with branches to the right and left to the kidneys and other organs in the abdomen, such as the stomach and liver. Since the kidneys must filter waste produces from the blood, they have an assured large supply, taking around one-fifth of the heart's output. Finally, the aorta sends a major artery into each leg. All over the body where there are arteries near the skin surface, the pressure wave caused by each heart beat can be felt as a pulse.

Arteries are essentially pipes for transporting blood, but they are not inflexible. Their walls are elastic, stretching with the surge of blood that accompanies each heart beat, and then contracting to maintain blood flow. If it were not for this recoil, blood could reach the most distant parts of the body only if it left the heart under enormous pressure. With old age, artery walls harden and begin to lose their elasticity. For this reason, blood pressure must increase to maintain the circulation.

Arteries enlarge under pressure of blood, but they also play an *active* role in regulating the circulation. The middle layer of an artery wall is a thick ring of muscle that can expand and contract, increasing or decreasing the diameter of the vessel and so controlling blood flow. Such control is essential since demand for blood in different parts of the body varies greatly according to our activity. With exercise, for example, supply to the major muscles must increase. (In many cases the demand for energy is ten or twenty times greater when muscle cells are active than when they are at rest.) After eating, blood is diverted to the gut so that nutrients are rapidly absorbed. When we overheat, blood is sent to the skin surface to cool, and kept away from it when we need to conserve heat. Even within the brain there are small but appreciable variations in blood flow as we perform different intellectual tasks. The arterial system adjusts to accommodate these changing needs.

Changes in artery diameter also influence overall blood pressure. If the arteries are narrow, the heart has to pump against a large resistance to the flow of blood, and the pressure is therefore greater. When arteries are relaxed, blood pressure falls. Muscles in the artery wall are largely under the control of the nervous system; and many of the drugs that affect blood pressure (*see* chapter 13) do so via their influence on this system.

Running roughly in parallel with the major arteries, but flowing in the opposite direction, are the veins that return blood to the heart. By the time blood reaches them, the pressure generated by the heart has been dissipated. Their walls are less thick and muscular than those of the arteries.

In someone who is standing, flow of blood back to the heart is largely against gravity. There must therefore be some force which propels blood along the veins. This force is provided by the action of the body's muscles. When our calf muscle contracts, for example, blood in the vein running through it comes under pressure. The effect is to squeeze blood upwards since valves at intervals along each vein prevent any downward flow – in much the same way that lock gates on a canal enable a boat to travel uphill. The valves' importance is shown most clearly when they fail, as is the case with varicose veins. Blood flows back down the vein, becoming pooled in the meandering sections of dilated blood vessel that form such a visible sign of this condition. In the abdomen, blood is concentrated in large veins before its return to the heart. Here, advantage is taken of the muscle movements accompanying breathing to shift the blood along.

The large blood vessels – the veins and arteries – are familiar enough, but they are not all that there is to the circulation. The real work of the blood is done in far smaller vessels, called the capillaries, which reach into every part of the body and ensure that none of our cells is more than a fraction of a millimetre away from a blood supply. Capillaries are so fine that many are smaller in diameter than individual red blood cells (which therefore have to 'deform' themselves to squeeze through). In total, we each contain around 40,000 miles of capillaries.

This intimate contact between blood and the cells it serves is necessary for the efficient exchange of gases, nutrients and waste products. Red blood cells, whose haemoglobin picked up oxygen so readily when the concentration of the gas was high in the small air sacs in the lungs, now lose it through the walls of the capillaries to cells that are poor in oxygen. By a reverse process, and in a fraction of a second, carbon dioxide diffuses from the tissues into the blood. When this blood returns to the lungs, carbon dioxide is exchanged for oxygen once more, and the carbon dioxide breathed out.

Blood pressure

Though raised blood pressure is a common medical problem, and increases the risk of stroke and certain kinds of heart disease, it is even more vital that the blood pressure does not become too low. Pressure is needed to keep blood in circulation, just as a 'head' of water in a tank is required to maintain the household water supply. Without adequate pressure, blood is not forced to move through the tissues (a process called perfusion) and there is no delivery of oxygen and nutrients.

We speak of 'blood pressure' in the singular, but there are in fact two blood pressures. Blood in the arteries is under higher pressure when the heart ventricles contract (systole) than when they are relaxed (diastole). Both pressures can be measured using the familiar arm cuff and stethoscope, giving a reading (as with atmospheric pressure) in millimetres (mm) of mercury. This represents the height that mercury would be forced to rise up a tube if arterial blood were flowing into one end of it. For a healthy young adult, an average systolic pressure is somewhere around 120 mm of mercury, though anywhere between 90 and 140 would be regarded as normal. An average diastolic pressure is around 80, with a range of 50–95 mm.

If the brain is deprived of oxygen for a few seconds, unconsciousness follows. A few minutes without it and the brain is dead. As the control centre of the body, the brain must therefore be well protected against loss of circulation. The body's blood pressure sensors are therefore located in the arteries that lead from the heart to the brain. At the first sign that blood pressure is falling below a critical point, counter-measures, such as the constriction of arteries, come into play.

Nevertheless, there are circumstances in which the heart rate slows, the blood vessels expand, blood drains from the head and the person faints. If this happens, the best response is to ensure that the head does not remain above the level of the rest of the body. This is usually achieved quite naturally when the person falls over. But people who faint in circumstances where they are kept upright (in toilet cubicles, for example) may die. The common and apparently helpful gesture of placing a collapsed person's head on a pillow is in fact counter-productive. It would be far better to raise their feet!

Chapter Two

What Can Go Wrong with the Heart?

We have talked about different aspects of the heart: its basic structure of four chambers, with major blood vessels connecting them to the body and lungs; the valves that control the direction in which blood flows; the muscle that powers the pump; the electrical system that sets heart rate and rhythm; and the small but crucial coronary arteries that supply the heart muscle itself with blood. Problems can occur with each of these elements. The diagnostic tests used to unravel exactly what is wrong are described in chapter 3, and the treatments for various forms of heart disease are then individually considered. For the moment we simply outline some general principles.

Birth defects

The heart begins its development as a single, slightly pulsating tube with arteries at one end and veins at the other. Within eight weeks of conception the tube has folded back on itself and developed the basic structures of the mature heart. Given the complexity of that organ, it is not surprising that the process occasionally goes wrong. Congenital heart defects (that is, those present at birth) are found in just under 1 per cent of babies. The use of ultrasound (or echo) scans, described in chapter 3, enables the heart of the fetus to be seen in sufficient detail at around 18 weeks for any defects to be apparent. In the unlikely event of a serious problem, doctors can then be ready at the birth to take immediate steps to save the baby's life.

The four heart chambers and two most important blood vessels can be thought of very simply as the six boxes shown in figure 2.1. When all is well, the six elements form in their proper place, and have the right connections with each other. But in the course of the heart's development in the womb, any number of different abnormal arrangements of these six elements can occur. For example, the right ventricle may develop where the left one should be: connected to the left atrium, and so receiving its blood not from the vessels returning from the body, but from the lungs. In other cases, the right ventricle may be in its proper place, but far too small; or there may be no division at all between the two beating chambers.

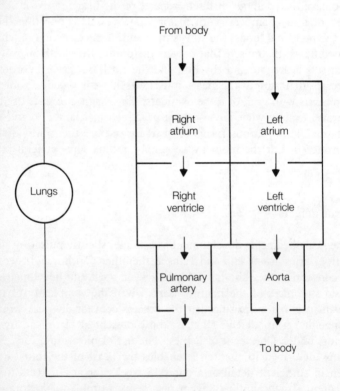

Figure 2.1 Six elements make up the normal heart and major blood vessels. In hearts that are defective at birth, any of these elements may be larger or smaller than normal, misplaced or missing altogether. Arrows show the dirction of blood flow.

Certain of these combinations make blood circulation impossible and cause death almost immediately; others can be tolerated for a while but must be corrected if the baby is to survive childhood. Where the abnormal connection means that blood re-circulates to the body without passing through the lungs, the baby will appear 'blue' from the colour of unoxygenated blood. 'Blue babies' may survive, but cannot take much exercise and their growth may be stunted unless the defect is corrected. Prompt surgery is also usually advised where the birth defect means that too *much* blood reaches the lungs. Although babies with this problem are not blue, their lungs may be damaged by the abnormally high flow and pressure of blood.

Among the conditions that reduce the heart's efficiency, but do not always cause major difficulty, are holes in the wall (called the septum) that separates the two sides of the heart. Holes between the collecting chambers (known as *atrial septal defects*) may be little problem, and stay undetected for years. Defects in the septum separating the ventricles are often more serious (especially where the lungs are placed at risk) and may require an operation to repair them, though some holes present at birth close of their own accord and others are too small to be significant.

Surgery for congenital heart defects is increasingly successful. It may still be necessary for a child to have two operations: initially to remedy the worst effects of the defect, and later to correct it completely. However, as the risk of such operations is reduced, the trend is towards complete correction at an earlier age. This limits disruption to the child's life, especially if all necessary surgery can be completed before school age. Early surgery also avoids potential damage and lessens the risk of heart infections, which are always possible when blood flow is turbulent. Infections due to congenital heart defects are rare before adolescence but may be a problem in later life.

There are figures and brief descriptions at the end of this chapter of some common forms of congenital heart defect.

Valve disease: narrowing and leakage

Blood is under greatest pressure when it is in the left ventricle since this heart chamber powers the circulation to all of the body except the lungs. Because of this pressure, the stresses imposed on both the mitral valve (separating left atrium and left ventricle) and the aortic valve (sealing the left ventricle from the body's major artery) are very great. These two valves are the ones that most frequently become diseased and may therefore require treatment and possible replacement; though the same difficulties also occur with the similar pair of valves on the right side of the heart.

Problems can arise either because the flaps of a valve become thickened and stiff and so obstruct the flow of blood (a condition called *stenosis*) or because the valve fails to shut properly and so stop blood flowing through it in the wrong direction. This leakage is known as *regurgitation*. The two problems often occur together. Both defects mean that blood does not move as it should through the heart: circulation of blood to the body is inadequate and organs work less efficiently.

The heart can compensate in various ways for the effects of damaged valves. However, as the condition worsens, symptoms may start to appear, either gradually or suddenly, depending on the valve affected and the precise problem involved. In many cases, the failing heart can be well supported using drugs. However, as the heart's ability to compensate declines, surgery may become necessary, and is best undertaken before there is irretrievable damage.

Valves may also stop working quite suddenly. One reason is rupture of the tendons (looking like parachute cords or guy ropes) that attach the leaflets of the mitral valve to the heart wall. Such events can catastrophically reduce blood circulation, and present a more immediate threat to life.

There are many causes of defective heart valves. In a few people, they are deformed before birth. This problem affects roughly one baby in 200 (though difficulties may not become apparent until late in life). In others, the valves are damaged as the result of a heart attack. Degeneration of heart valves due to simple wear and tear is also increasingly recognised as a source of problems in our growing elderly population. But the most common cause of valve disease is still the legacy of rheumatic fever (described below in the section on infections) which leads to gradual deterioration of the valves over decades. Chapter 8 describes how heart valve disease is treated.

Very rarely, the mitral valve is narrowed not by disease of the valve itself but by an abnormal growth in the atrium. Unlike many other tumours, such growths (termed *myxomas*) are generally not malignant and are removed by surgery.

Coronary artery disease: 'hardening of the arteries'

Almost all middle-aged and elderly people in Western societies have arteries that are affected by a disease called *atherosclerosis*. In this condition, a mixture of fat and fibrous blood components (known as *atheroma*) starts to accumulate along blood vessel walls. The result is hardening of the arterial wall (hence the term 'sclerosis'), gradual obstruction of the vessel, and so reduced flow of blood.

In the aorta, signs of the condition appear in males around adolescence. The first deposits are actually inside cells and form 'fatty streaks' that do not obstruct the smooth internal lining of the artery. But with early middle age (and about two decades later in women), a different form of deposit starts to occur. Now the fat forms raised, rough encrustations that may appreciably narrow the diameter of the artery. This is especially so with the smaller blood vessels such as the coronary arteries (shown in figure 1.8).

We have spoken so far of fat, and a major component of the lumpy, yellowish deposit is cholesterol and its many compounds. But atheroma also contains cells: red blood cells, suggesting there has been bleeding into the deposit, and white cells, which take part in the process of inflammation and are normally employed in fighting infection. There is also a fibrous 'scaffolding', consisting of the fibrin strands that are the basis of blood clotting, along which the deposit seems to grow.

As for the origins of atheroma, it may be that fats in the blood-stream become absorbed into the artery wall. This explanation suggests diet as a major cause of the disease. (The role of cholesterol is discussed in chapter 12). On the other hand, the varied ingredients of the deposited 'porridge' (the Greek word for porridge gives us the term 'atheroma') suggest a more complicated explanation.

With time, atheroma becomes hardened by the addition of calcium deposits. This makes the encrustations brittle. If they split, pieces may break off and swirl away in the blood to block vessels further downstream where they become lodged, a problem known as *embolism*. Where raw artery wall is exposed, blood will tend to clot. The clots formed (they are also called *thrombus*) may grow to block the blood vessel at the place where the plaque is ruptured; or may again be carried off to cause an obstruction elsewhere.

These processes (figure 2.2) can occur in all arteries. When the obstruction they cause is in the brain, a stroke ensues. (Blocked

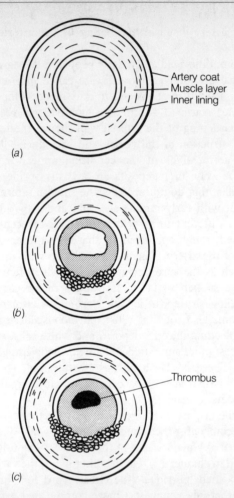

Figure 2.2 'Hardening of the arteries': the development of atheroma. (*a*)
Cross-section through a healthy artery. (*b*) Fatty substances, including
cholesterol, are deposited in the lining of the artery along with blood
platelets, and muscle cells grow in from the middle layer. The process may
start at a point where the lining of the artery is damaged, but soon becomes
widespread. As the deposit (called 'plaque' or atheroma) ages, it acts as a
focus for the formation of blood clots. Calcium is deposited and the
atheroma becomes stiff and brittle, preventing the blood vessel from dilating
as well as reducing its diameter. (*c*) The artery finally becomes completely
blocked as a blood clot (thrombus) forms.

arteries are one of the causes of stroke. The other important cause is bursting of an artery, which damages brain tissue first by the initial explosive force of the rupture, and then by the swelling that follows). Where tiny blood vessels in the eye are blocked, a small area of retina dies and a blind spot develops. Obstruction of arteries in the fingers, toes, arms and legs reduces oxygen supply to distant parts of the body and if severe enough may lead to the death of skin and muscle, the development of gangrene and perhaps the need for amputation. In the heart, complete obstruction of the coronary arteries leads to death of part of the heart muscle during a heart attack.

Blockage of an artery by a clot (or thrombus) in the way described is a sudden event. But it is clear that the process leading up to it is gradual. If it were not for the slow narrowing of arteries by atheroma, clots would have fewer opportunities to form and fewer sites at which to block blood flow. It is also clear that fatty deposits in the arterial wall may become so thick that the blood vessel is effectively blocked even without the contribution of a clot.

Heart attack and angina

In a heart attack, passage of blood down the affected artery ceases; and the area of heart muscle served by that artery dies over a period of hours if supplies of blood – and therefore of oxygen – are not restored. Heart muscle cannot regrow. The affected area of heart may heal, in the sense that a scar of dead tissue forms; but it never again takes part in the work of the heart. When a large area of muscle is lost, the pumping capacity of the heart is therefore seriously weakened. Reduced output of blood means less oxygen and nutrition for the tissues (including the heart itself) and can produce a downward spiral leading to heart failure. When 40 per cent or more of heart muscle is lost, the risk of heart failure is greatly increased. There may also be difficulties if smaller but critically sited areas of muscle are affected. These problems are discussed in chapter 4.

As explained in chapter 1, the work of the left ventricle is the most important to the circulation. It is here that heart muscle is thickest and the demand for blood greatest. The left ventricle is also the part most likely to experience a heart attack.

In a heart attack, coronary blood vessels become completely blocked, and little or no oxygen gets through to the muscle. But heart muscle may start to suffer even when there is no blockage, if its blood supply is so restricted that the demand for oxygen regularly exceeds its supply. An imbalance between supply and demand is especially likely when a person is taking exercise, since the heart is then having to work at maximum capacity. Heart muscle that is deprived of blood is unable to contribute effectively to pumping performance. A person's ability to exercise is therefore reduced. Often the restriction in blood supply leads to pain: the characteristic chest pain of angina.

Heart attacks and angina are therefore two aspects of the same disease. Since lack of blood is called *ischaemia*, the underlying condition is known as *ischaemic heart disease*.

Problems with heart muscle

Any pump requires power, provided in this case by the muscle of the heart wall. In most circumstances, as we have just seen, the major threat to heart muscle is from lack of oxygen. The problem may arise suddenly and catastrophically (in the case of some heart attacks), in stages (following a series of small heart attacks) or progressively over many years as the heart muscle is damaged by being forced to work with indequate supplies of fuel.

Apart from the problem of coronary artery disease, the heart muscle – known as the *myocardium* – can be damaged by viruses and bacteria (*see* the section below on infections). It is also subject to certain disorders which seem to affect the myocardium and nothing else. These diseases are called *cardiomyopathies*.

In some people, the muscle fibres of the heart wall grow too thick, reducing the volume of the heart chambers and eventually obstructing the proper flow of blood out of it. In others, the opposite occurs: the heart muscle becomes flabby and weak, the heart chambers distend and the ventricles pump with reduced force. This problem may occur as a late complication months or years after infection by viruses, but in other cases the cause is unknown. Progressive heart failure from these forms of cardiomyopathy can only be cured by heart transplantation, and the occurrence of the disease in young people is a major reason for the operation.

Abnormal heart rates and rhythms

If the heart beats too slowly, pressure in the circulation falls, insufficient blood reaches the brain and a person loses consciousness. The same problem can occur when the heart beats abnormally fast, since there is too little time for the heart chambers to fill with blood before they contract. To circulate blood effectively, heart rate must therefore be kept within limits, though these are wide (ranging from around 50 beats per minute to 150 or more).

When the normal pacemaker in the atrium is damaged or becomes disconnected from the rest of the electrical circuit, small centres in other parts of the heart take over. Though they usually set it beating at a slower rate, these fall-back pacemakers are an effective safeguard against the heart stopping altogether.

Other electrical problems can be caused by forms of short-circuit in the heart's conduction system. Instead of spreading in the normal, controlled way, current may (for example) bypass the relay station between atria and ventricles, firing the beating chambers too early in the heart cycle. The circuitry that keeps the heart beating in a coordinated way is shown in figure 1.6. Problems that affect it, and how they are dealt with, form the subject of chapter 7.

Infections

Infections of the heart, whether caused by bacteria or viruses, are rare, but when they occur they may have serious consequences. People who already have heart abnormalities (such as congenital defects and diseased or artificial valves) are at greater risk of heart infections than those with a healthy heart.

If we imagine a cross-section through the wall of the heart, we can distinguish three layers of tissue. The inner lining, including the heart valves, is called the *endocardium*; then comes the muscle mass of the heart, the *myocardium*; and finally the fibrous sac (*pericardium*) that encloses the heart. Each of these three layers may become infected and inflamed.

Infection of the heart valves: endocarditis

Endocarditis is the term used for infections of the heart valves and the tissue that lines the heart chambers.

Any disease-causing bacteria that enter the blood can infect the heart. There are probably small numbers of infective organisms passing through it all the time, causing no harm. But when flow of blood is sluggish or turbulent, and where the inner surfaces of the heart are uneven, bacteria may be able to gain a foothold and form colonies. This can happen around a damaged valve or hole in the heart, for example. Cells and blood products and then bacteria accumulate, forming irregular deposits (called vegetations). The difficulty usually arises in hearts that are already abnormal because of a previous infection, birth defect, surgery or simply the wear-and-tear of ageing. Any artificial surfaces formed by mechanical heart valves and by patches used to repair holes in the heart also increase the risk of bacterial infection.

The danger is obviously greatest when someone is exposed to unusually large numbers of bacteria. Even minor surgical procedures such as dental fillings and extractions allow bacteria easy entry to the blood. For this reason, people with certain kinds of heart problem are given antibiotics before and after a visit to the dentist to make sure that any exposure to bacteria will be controlled. Though bacteria are the usual cause of endocarditis, tiny fungi are also capable of causing infection.

Many heart infections are difficult to diagnose. A person feels unwell, and perhaps has a fever without an obvious cause. But there are few specific signs and symptoms of endocarditis; and much of the damage caused (such as holes and scars that further affect the efficiency of heart valves) is gradual.

Quick identification of endocarditis is important since infections at an early stage can often be cured by antibiotics, usually given by intravenous injection directly into the blood to ensure a better effect. When the infection is not cured, there is a danger of emboli: sudden blockage of blood vessels by pieces of infected vegetation that break off the heart valves and circulate in the blood until they become lodged in a small vessel in organs such as the brain and kidney. Where this is a risk, surgery may be advisable to remove infected parts of the heart. Endocarditis can also destroy heart valves, leading to severe heart failure and requiring urgent replacement of the valve by surgery.

Infection of the heart muscle: myocarditis

Infection of the heart muscle by bacteria is very rare, but the myocardium may be infected by viruses in the same way that any muscle of the body can be affected by a flu-like illness. Probably most of us have had viral infections of the heart muscle that have passed unnoticed. But, in a small number of cases, such infection causes severe damage and leads to gradual failure of the pumping capacity of the heart.

Infection of the heart sac: pericarditis

The sac that surrounds the heart (the pericardium) is occasionally infected by bacteria, and more frequently by viruses. Such infection is the most common cause of a build-up of fluid between the sac and the heart itself (though this problem may also arise following a heart attack). Accumulation of fluid increases pressure on the heart and restricts its ability to fill effectively, so reducing its pumping ability.

In the past, tuberculosis (TB) was a common cause of pericarditis, but it is now rare in the developed world. TB also led to thickening of the sac and the accumulation of calcium deposits that constricted heart movement so severely that the pericardium had to be cut away by surgery.

Rheumatic fever

As late as the 1930s, the most important threat to the heart was rheumatic fever, which affected more than one child in ten. Many children went on to develop heart valve problems that led – years later – to heart failure. Rheumatic fever follows infection (usually of the throat) by streptococcus bacteria. However, it does not appear until the infection itself has disappeared. And its cause is not the bacteria themselves, but the body's defensive response: antibodies are produced that cross-react with the structure of the heart.

The result is progressive damage, especially to the heart valves. Most people affected eventually need drug treatment; and, in many cases, replacement of the heart valves is the best course. When this is needed, surgery should take place early enough in the development of the disease for the operation to have a good chance of success. The mitral and aortic valves, on the left side of the heart, are the most likely to be affected. The problems caused have already been outlined, and we return to their treatment in chapter 8.

People with rheumatic heart disease run greater risks of the heart infections described earlier in this section. There is also a greater chance that abnormalities will develop in the heart muscle and in its conduction system. Rheumatic fever is one of the common causes, for example, of atrial fibrillation (*see* chapter 7).

Partly as a result of improved social conditions and partly because of effective antibiotics, rheumatic fever now occurs in fewer than one in 5,000 children. Fifteen years ago, the bulk of heart surgery involved replacing heart valves damaged by rheumatic disease. Though the problem continues in the developing world, it is now less prevalent in Europe and North America.

Some congenital heart defects

The first part of this chapter explained the way the heart is formed and how the process occasionally goes wrong. We here consider certain problems in greater detail.

There is a very slight tendency for congenital heart disorders to run in families, but it is very unlikely that a child will be born with a congenital defect even when a brother or sister has experienced the problem. As with all birth defects, exposure to the German measles virus early in pregnancy increases the risk of heart abnormalities.

Many birth abnormalities cure themselves. For example, half the 'holes in the heart' present at birth close of their own accord; and the majority of the 5,000 babies born in Britain each year with heart defects do not need surgery. In the 2,000 who do, the problem is corrected in 80 per cent of cases and improved in most of the others. Heart defects present at birth are one of many causes of slow growth and development or 'failure to thrive'. When this happens, repair of the defect usually results in a growth spurt in which the child catches up lost ground.

Surgery for simple congenital heart defects carries very little risk, but any complicated operation is obviously associated with a greater mortality. In the first few months of life, the risk of babies dying from surgery is higher, partly because only the most serious defects are operated on at this very early stage. Risks decrease in babies who have surgery towards the age of one year, and in those who are older than that the average chance of death from an operation to correct a congenital heart defect is around one in twenty.

Congenital heart defects occur in seven babies out of every 1,000 born alive. The most common congenital defect is a hole in the wall between the left and right ventricles: a condition called *ventricular*

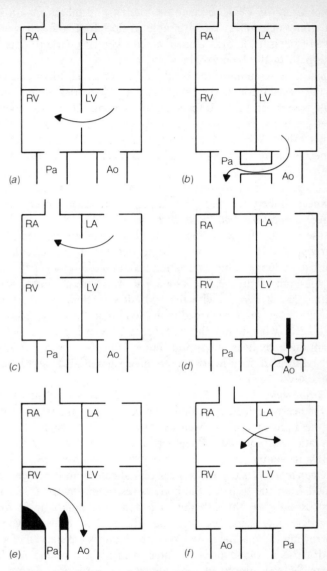

Figure 2.3 Six common heart defects found at birth: (*a*) ventricular septal defect; (*b*) persistent ductus arteriosus; (*c*) atrial septal defect; (*d*) coarctation of the aorta; (*e*) tetralogy of Fallot; (*f*) transposition of the great arteries. The last two produce 'blue babies'. A full explanation is given in text. RA/LA, right/left atrium; RV/LV, right/left ventricle; Ao, aorta; Pa, pulmonary artery.

septal defect (or VSD). Because the pumping chambers are not sealed off from each other, blood is able to flow from the left ventricle (where pressure is high) into the right ventricle (where it is low). The path of the blood is shown by an arrow in figure 2.3*a*. If the defect is large enough, the result is that too much blood passes out of the heart through the pulmonary artery to the lungs; and too little is pumped through the aorta and around the body. Blood that does get to the body has passed through the lungs, and so the baby is not 'blue'. When a baby's only problem is a VSD, surgery (if it is needed at all) carries little risk. VSDs are found in two babies of every 1,000 born.

In about half that number of babies the problem is an abnormal connection between the aorta and the pulmonary artery: a birth defect called *persistent ductus arteriosus* (or PDA). When the baby is in the womb, the aorta and pulmonary artery are connected. The purpose of this short-circuit is to prevent blood from circulating to the baby's lungs. This connection should close up at birth. Where it does not (figure 2.3*b*), blood passes from the aorta into the pulmonary artery. As with the VSD described above, the result is that the lungs are overloaded with blood, and the body receives too little. But what blood the body does receive is oxygen-rich, and again the baby does not appear 'blue'. Surgery to close a PDA does not require an open-heart operation (*see* appendix 1) and is usually not risky.

Atrial septal defects are holes between the two collecting chambers of the heart (figure 2.3*c*), allowing blood to pass from the left atrium to the right atrium, as well as into the left ventricle. Often, no operation is required. When repair is needed, surgery to correct ASDs in young children is unlikely to cause problems.

Coarctation of the aorta is a congenital condition in which flow of blood from the heart to the body is restricted (figure 2.3*d*). Blood that cannot pass through the narrowed aorta builds up in the left ventricle, increasing pressure and straining the heart. Beyond the narrowing there is too little blood, the kidneys are starved of supply and a rise in blood pressure later in life is a common result if a normal blood supply to the kidneys is not restored. Surgery for coarctation of the aorta does not involve an open-heart operation and is regarded as simple by today's standards.

The most common cause of 'blue babies' is a condition called *tetralogy of Fallot*, which is found once in every 2,000 births. Here, there is a combination of four distinct defects, including excessive growth of muscle in the right ventricle and a large hole between the heart's pumping chambers (ventricular septal defect). This problem, combined with an abnormally large aorta and an abnormally narrow exit to the pulmonary artery, allows unoxygenated blood to circulate from the right ventricle to the body without first flowing through the lungs. The path of blood is shown by the arrow in figure 2.3*e*. The result is that the baby appears cyanosed (i.e. blue). Babies with tetralogy of Fallot are successfully operated upon; but the challenge is greater than for the simpler defects considered so far.

A second cause of 'blue babies' is *transposition of the great arteries*, in which the aorta is attached to the right ventricle and the pulmonary artery to the left ventricle, instead of the reverse (figure 2.3*f*). Babies with this condition can survive only if there is an abnormal connection somewhere between the two circulations. Most often this connection takes the form of a hole between the atria. Without this mixing of blood, the two circulations (to the lungs and to the body) would be entirely separate, and the body would receive no oxygenated blood at all. Transposition is a complicated form of congenital defect, but can still be successfully corrected by surgery.

Chapter Three

Diagnosing Heart Disease

Many people who seek a specialist's opinion do not have significant heart disease. Some may have minor heart problems that pose no real threat; some may have symptoms that suggest heart disease but that actually arise from other organs in the body; and others may have little wrong with them at all. A cardiologist uses skill and experience to identify and help those people who have important problems – and reassures the rest.

The information that a doctor gathers starts with a 'history', the patient's description of symptoms: what they feel like, when they were first experienced and how they have changed with time. This is followed by a physical examination, during which the doctor looks for signs of disease that may not have been noticed by the patient.

With certain heart disorders, such as narrowing of the mitral valve, increasingly severe symptoms and signs parallel the progress of the disease. With other problems, and especially with the silting up of the blood vessels that fuel the heart, there may be no obvious indications that anything is wrong until late in the development of the disease. Crucial coronary arteries can be three-quarters blocked and still produce no chest pain, for example. Often enough (in fact, in around one-third of cases), the first indication that a patient or his doctor has of coronary artery disease is the heart attack itself.

As we become more concerned about screening patients who do not have symptoms, and are able to use increasingly sophisticated aids to diagnosis, this position is beginning to change. One of the most important developments in the early detection and treatment of coronary artery disease is the exercise ECG, explained below. But an examination by the doctor will still start with simple questions about symptoms, whether or not heart disease is suspected and whatever the form of the disease may be.

As with any illness, heart problems can cause many very general problems such as extreme sleepiness, lack of energy and feelings of being unwell. People who have had a heart attack often say it was preceded by weeks or months of increasing fatigue. However, there are more specific symptoms.

Symptoms of heart disease

Breathlessness

Unusual shortness of breath – sufficient to interfere with everyday activities – is a frequent indication that the heart is not working well, though breathlessness can have other causes, such as lung disease and anaemia. This symptom (called *dyspnoea*) may be felt as a need to breathe more deeply or to take extra breaths; it may affect a person only when active – perhaps climbing the stairs – or also when resting. Some people experience particular problems when lying flat, and so sleep with extra pillows to prevent themselves waking up short of breath during the night. People who think that they are more breathless than they should be (given their age, fitness and degree of physical activity) would be wise to consult a doctor.

Pain

Chest pain is an uncomfortable and immediately disquieting symptom. If it is felt in the centre of the body as a crushing sensation, spreads to the arms and neck and if it is accompanied by sweating and a feeling of nausea, then the heart is likely to be the cause, though there are many other problems (some of them minor) that also produce chest pain. Whatever the reason, severe discomfort in the chest is a clear indication that a doctor should be consulted. The pain or discomfort of angina and the pain felt during a heart attack are described in detail in chapters 4 and 6.

Palpitations

Although the heart is a powerful pump, it is a surprising fact that for most of the time we remain unaware of it. Clearly, there are the usual circumstances, such as fright, excitement and exercise, when

we are conscious of its efforts. When someone is aware of their
heart in other, abnormal situations, the sensation may suggest heart
problems. Sometimes it is as if the heart stops briefly, restarting
again with a powerful thump; at other times, the awareness is of
the heart beating more slowly than normal, or faster – like a
fluttering in the chest – but without any obvious cause. Such palpitations (which can be either regular or irregular) may be a symptom of heart disease and should be checked, though most are found
to have quite innocent causes.

Fainting

Dizziness and fainting occur when the brain is deprived of sufficient
blood. People faint for many reasons: usually they have nothing to
do with the heart. Nevertheless, fainting and dizziness can be
the first symptoms of certain kinds of valve disease, and are also
experienced when the heart beats abnormally fast or slowly. The
most usual cause, however, is a fall in blood pressure brought about
(for example) by standing for too long or getting too quickly out of
a hot bath, in which case they are not an indication of serious
disease. The medical term for sudden fainting, or loss of consciousness, is *syncope*.

When the heart is not beating with a normal rhythm, or is in
some other way working inefficiently, symptoms of an inadequate
circulation may develop. In addition to the spells of light-
headedness, dizziness and fainting already mentioned, symptoms of
poor circulation include unusual coldness in the hands and feet and
swelling around the ankles.

Swelling

When it cannot pump enough blood, the heart acts like a dam,
causing a build-up of blood in the veins. Fluid leaks out of the
blood vessels and gathers at the feet under force of gravity, a
condition called *oedema*. In addition to ankle swelling, enlargement
of the stomach and a tender liver, and expansion of veins in the
neck are signs that the heart is failing to circulate blood effectively.
All are caused by the damming back of blood unable to return to
the heart.

Signs of heart disease

The patient's account of why he or she thinks there may be something wrong is vital information. The doctor's physical examination adds to this, and includes the following features.

Pulse

The pulse provides evidence about heart rate and the regularity of its rhythm. The volume of the pulse (whether it is weak and 'thready' or full and 'bounding') indicates the state of the circulation. The experienced observer may also be able to tell from the quality of the pulse something about the state of the aortic valve.

The inside of the wrist is an obvious point to take the pulse, but the body has many other places where a pulse can be felt. These include the inside of the forearm at the elbow, either groin, behind the knees, at the ankles and in the neck. Pulses that occur later than they should, or that are weak or missing, provide information about obstructions in the circulation.

Blood pressure

When the heart contracts (called *systole*), blood in the body's arteries is at higher pressure than when the beating chambers relax (*diastole*). Measurement of blood pressure therefore gives two values: systolic and diastolic. In the traditional method of blood pressure measurement, a cuff is placed around the upper arm and inflated until the artery beneath is squashed flat, preventing any flow of blood. The pressure in the cuff is then gradually released until spurting noises heard through the stethoscope show that blood has begun to pass through again. At this point, blood flows through intermittently, only when the heart contracts. This is therefore the systolic pressure. Only when the pressure in the cuff is released further will the blood start to flow also when the heart is in its relaxed phase. The point at which this continuous flow starts shows the diastolic pressure. In modern monitors, detection of the two pressures is automatic and a digital read-out gives the two values. However, the principle is the same as in the older instruments (called sphygmomanometers) with the mercury-filled tubes.

As with all signs and symptoms, blood pressure must always be considered in the context of the other pieces in the diagnostic jigsaw. In some patients, high blood pressure – a condition called *hypertension* – suggests the presence of a particular disease; but in many others there is no identifiable cause. Such high blood pressure is termed 'essential', which is simply an admission that we do not know why it occurs. However, it may still be important to treat the condition, in the hope that damage to the arteries will be reduced and the risk of stroke and heart attack reduced (*see* chapter 12).

Blood pressure varies greatly from one person to another, and in any individual it changes through the day and according to stress and physical activity. So there is a wide spread of readings that can be regarded as normal. But many people have blood pressures that are consistently out of this range; and both high and low readings can alert the doctor to the presence of disease. For example, unusually low blood pressure may be a sign of heart failure or obstruction in the heart valves; and a large difference between the systolic and diastolic values could indicate a leaking aortic valve.

'Feeling' the heart

Doctors can obtain some information about the heart by feeling its beat against the chest wall. If the heart is enlarged, the prominent beat at its tip is felt in an abnormal position. (This usually means the left ventricle is affected.) If the right ventricle is unusually big, the doctor's hand can detect an abnormal pulsation on the front of the chest wall. Certain disturbances of heart rhythm can also be felt by laying a hand on the chest.

Heart sounds

The stethoscope is simply a tool to amplify sound. It was first designed by the Frenchman Laennec in 1816, and is said to have had tubes 3 feet long, because that was a distance greater than a flea could jump. Apart from being shorter, and having a flat rather than a conical end, the stethoscope has not changed since then.

Noises the heart makes reveal much about its condition. The 'lub-dup' of the healthy heartbeat is the sound of heart valves closing. The stethoscope therefore provides important information about their activity. There are other, less important, noises; but a particular feature of certain unhealthy hearts is the presence of murmurs (rushing and swishing sounds) caused by turbulence in the blood as it passes through damaged valves or holes in the heart wall. There are many murmurs whose position, quality of sound and pitch provide clear evidence of certain kinds of abnormality. Not all murmurs signify disease, though; and murmurs that are loud are not necessarily worse than those that are soft. In children, for example, very small holes between the beating chambers can cause considerable turbulence in the blood and so produce a loud murmur, and yet be unimportant.

Breath sounds

The stethoscope is also used to listen to sounds from the lungs. A heart which is not working well leads to the build-up of fluid, producing stiffness in the lungs, and crackles and wheezy sounds as the air moves in and out. To the patient, the problem is evident as breathlessness.

Special tests

A normal person is only someone who has not been adequately investigated – or so it has been said. The element of truth here is that many perfectly healthy people show peculiarities of heart function (particularly of heart rhythm) that are not related to disease and are nothing to worry about. The results of a particular test, considered on their own, may therefore mean very little. But if the physical examination turns up any suggestion of a problem, more detailed investigation is desirable.

X-Rays

The most general of these investigations is a chest X-ray, taken from the back and sides if the heart is being examined, and always with the patient standing in the same position so that X-rays from different occasions can be compared.

The heart appears on an X-ray as a shadow. Very occasionally, both doctor and patient are surprised to find the heart is on the right of the chest (which is a completely harmless variation from the normal). But interest usually centres on the size and shape of the shadow, since both can provide clues about the presence of disease. The shadow represents not just the heart itself, but also the first sections of two important blood vessels (the aorta and pulmonary artery) and the fibrous sac that surrounds the heart. Usually, the sac wraps the heart closely around, but there may be fluid present, in which case it expands and makes the shadow appear larger.

On occasions, an X-ray reveals direct evidence that chalky calcium deposits have been laid down within the heart or the major blood vessels. The X-ray appearance of the lungs is also important since the pattern of blood flow in its major vessels and the presence of fluid may provide evidence of heart failure.

Asking the patient to swallow barium, a harmless substance which can easily be seen on X-rays, outlines the oesophagus (gullet) behind the heart. This simple investigation was once much used to help the doctor decide whether the heart was enlarged, and if so, which chambers were abnormal. Barium X-rays are now used less frequently because of the information provided by ultrasound (*see* below).

The ECG (EKG)

Described as the electrical signature of the heart, the electrocardiogram (ECG) was first recorded by Willem Einthoven in 1903. Traditionally, the ECG has been the doctor's most valuable technical aid in diagnosing heart disease. It provides the first clear evidence of whether or not there has been a heart attack, and allows instant diagnosis of the many abnormalities of heart rhythm, certain of which require urgent treatment. More recent developments in ECG technique also tell us whether the heart muscle is dangerously deprived of blood, and so provide the opportunity for heart attacks to be prevented. The ECG records the very small amounts of electricity (measured in millivolts) produced by the collecting and beating chambers of the heart as they repeatedly contract and relax. It is obtained by placing electrodes at different points on the chest, and on the arms and legs. By varying the position of the electrodes (there can be as many as twelve), electrical activity in different areas of the heart can be assessed. Apart from the application of jelly to the skin (to aid electrical conduction) the patient feels nothing. No electricity flows into the body, and the procedure is entirely painless.

The record of the heart's electrical activity appears as the familiar wavy line on a piece of moving graph paper or on a small TV screen

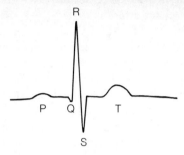

Figure 3.1 A typical ECG trace showing the electrical activity during a single heart beat. Each characteristic up or down deflection (called a wave) is referred to by a letter.

(figure 3.1). Electrical current moving through the heart towards the recording electrode produces an upward deflection on the trace, and current moving away a downward deflection. (The 'circuitry' in the heart that is responsible is described in chapter 1.)

The most straightforward information given by the ECG is the rate at which the heart is beating. The graph paper on a standard ECG machine moves at a speed of five large squares per second so that the frequency of the heart beat (taken as the interval between the large peaks) can easily be calculated. The ECG also reveals the heart's rhythm, showing whether it is working in a coordinated or uncoordinated way. We can learn about the state of the conduction system that controls pumping, since the ECG shows how electrical signals travel through heart muscle; and the size of the heart can be estimated from the amount of electrical activity it produces.

Events such as heart attacks, which leave a permanent scar in the heart muscle, generally also leave a characteristic imprint on the ECG trace. The location of these areas of dead heart muscle can be pinpointed. However, with small heart attacks, the ECG changes that usually occur soon after the event may later disappear.

Exercise ECG

The ECG can be a versatile and invaluable way of finding out something of the history of the heart and its current condition. But the standard ECG – recorded with the patient at rest – is not particularly good at telling us what the future holds. In particular, the ECG trace can appear quite normal even when there is severe disease in the coronary arteries.

For this reason, the exercise ECG (also called simply the exercise test or 'stress test') is now becoming important in the diagnosis of coronary artery disease. In this test, a patient gradually increases his or her level of physical activity while the ECG is continuously recorded. This may involve an adapted bicycle or a small section of steps. But the most usual technique is to have the patient walk on a moving belt (or treadmill) as its speed and slope are slowly increased. To standardise conditions from one test to another, a routine procedure is followed. In the most common protocol (called the Bruce test), the patient starts by walking for 1 minute at just under 2 miles an hour on the level, followed by 3 minutes at the same speed with a gradient of one in ten, 3 minutes at 2.5 mph with a gradient of 12 per cent, and so on.

Anyone who can walk can have an exercise ECG: it does not require an athlete's level of fitness. What is important is not how 'well' someone does, but the information the test provides about the condition of his or her heart.

The exercise test is safe, since changes in the ECG (and usually also in blood pressure) are closely monitored. But placing the heart under this controlled amount of stress can reveal areas of muscle that are receiving inadequate amounts of blood because of obstructions in the coronary arteries. The technique is therefore good at establishing which patients are at risk of a heart attack. This allows time for the problem to be investigated further and, it is hoped, to enable doctors to start treatment that will prevent the heart attack.

In chapter 6 we describe the usefulness of exercise tests in deciding the best treatment for angina. The exercise ECG is also helpful in diagnosing certain abnormalities of heart rhythm that occur only when a person exercises. Stress tests (usually starting with a very mild degree of exercise) are valuable in patients who are recovering from a heart attack. If they are negative (that is, no ECG abnormalities are detected), the patient knows he can exercise to that point without risk to the heart. Self-confidence therefore increases. Exercise tests that are positive after a heart attack show that significant problems remain with the supply of blood to the heart muscle. This may suggest that treatment (perhaps with drugs or surgery) is needed.

24-hour ECG

Another valuable refinement of ECG technology is continuous recording of the heart's electrical activity over a period of 24 hours as the patient goes about his usual life. This 'ambulatory' monitoring provides evidence about occasional disturbances of heart rhythm that are otherwise difficult to detect. Though they may not happen often in the course of a day, such rhythm irregularities can be dangerous enough to require treatment. ECG monitoring over 24 hours also shows whether areas of heart muscle are periodically being deprived of oxygen. During this Holter recording (named after the American physicist who pioneered the technique), the patient is fitted out with a convenient, small, portable ECG machine which records the heart's electrical activity on tape cassettes.

Echo (ultrasound) scans

Ultrasound is a widely used diagnostic technique, pioneered by doctors who needed a safe way of following the development of the fetus during pregnancy. Its application to cardiology (called *echocardiography*) provides another safe and painless way of finding out about the heart's form and function. The ultrasound principle lies behind underwater sonar used to locate submarines or shoals of fish: in the medical context, high-frequency sound waves are bounced off structures such as those in the heart. The record of their return gives a cross-sectional image showing size, 'depth' and density. A small device (called a transducer) placed against the skin of the chest and pointed at the heart both emits the ultrasound waves and acts as a receiver.

The essence of the heart's function is that it never stands still. Since echo traces show changes that occur with time (valves as they open and close, for example), they are particularly helpful in cardiology. One form of echocardiography, called M-Mode, produces a complicated 'one-dimensional' trace. More recent 2-D echo gives us cross-sectional pictures of the heart and film and video images in which its beating chambers and moving valves can clearly be seen. From these traces and images, doctors can measure the thickness of the ventricle walls, tell whether they contract in a coordinated way and establish whether the heart valves open as freely and close as tightly as they should. Ultrasound also reveals any build-up of fluid around the heart and the lungs.

Because echo is entirely safe, and relatively cheap (the equipment costs £30,000–80,000 and each scan around £50), it is increasingly used to check on the progress of disease, and to monitor the effects of treatment. 2-D is also becoming widely accepted as the best way of diagnosing congenital defects. In women who are 20 weeks pregnant, the fetus' heart is less than 1 centimetre across. Yet 2-D echo is capable of identifying most abnormalities that occur.

Using catheters: diagnosis from inside the heart

Despite the wealth of information about the heart that can be obtained from outside the body, there are times when more is needed. For this reason, safe methods of inserting diagnostic instruments into the heart itself have been developed. Their use means doctors can establish with far greater certainty where any problems lie, and so plan more effective treatment.

There is a variety of techniques, but all involve a similar procedure. After the patient has been given a mild sedative and a local anaesthetic, a long, fine, flexible tube is inserted into a vein or artery in the arm or groin. (This involves either a very small surgical cut or puncturing the blood vessel with a fine needle.) The tube is then delicately pushed along the blood vessel until it reaches the heart. Where the aim is to reach the right side of the heart and the lungs, a vein is used for the approach; for the left side of the heart, an artery.

The narrow tube is called a *catheter*, and the procedure *cardiac catheterisation*. Catheters do two closely linked jobs. First, they obtain direct information about the way the heart is working: about how much blood it is actually pumping, for example. Secondly, they enable doctors to use X-rays to provide more detailed images of the heart. So catheters provide evidence about heart structure as well as function.

It was in 1929 that a young German doctor called Forssmann first demonstrated that a catheter could reach the human heart. He did so not with the help of a patient but – against explicit orders – by catheterising himself! Standing behind an X-ray screen so that an image was produced of his chest, Forssmann watched its reflection in a mirror as he slowly manoeuvred the catheter into his heart. Despite his success, the technique was initially frowned upon. But 30 years later its wide usefulness was recognised, and Forssmann (together with an American and Frenchman who further developed the technique) were awarded a Nobel prize.

Now, almost everyone who is to have heart surgery will first have their hearts studied using a catheter. However, procedures are changing, and other, less 'invasive' techniques (such as echocardiography) are increasingly used to make decisions about future care. Whatever the method, the important consideration is that the surgeon knows exactly where any problem lies. Cardiac catheterisation may cause some discomfort but does not usually cause any pain. A catheter in a blood vessel or in the heart rarely produces any sensation. Though catheter studies are a normal prelude to surgery, clearly not everyone who is investigated with a catheter will need a heart operation.

Catheters to measure pressure, blood output and oxygen

Catheters can be used to measure pressures within the heart's chambers and the major blood vessels, recording the way they vary at different stages in the beating cycle. Departures from the expected pattern may reflect the failure of valves to open or shut properly, or defects in pumping performance.

The amount of blood being pumped by the heart (the cardiac output) can be estimated by injecting small quantities of dye or cold fluid and measuring the speed with which the material becomes diluted as it passes through the heart.

If it is suspected that there may be abnormal connections between the chambers of the heart, a slightly different approach is called for. A catheter is moved through the heart to measure the concentration of oxygen at different points. The sudden appearance of oxygen-rich blood from the lungs in the right side of the heart, which normally contains only the oxygen-depleted blood returning from the circulation, is evidence of a tear or hole in one of the internal walls. Similar abnormal connections between the heart chambers may cause the sudden appearance of oxygen-depleted blood where it should not be found.

Catheters to record rhythm and conduction

Certain irregularities of heart beat are best studied by inserting yet another type of catheter, through which electrical activity in the heart is measured. The technique is called electrophysiology. The information provided by an ECG, where the electrodes are on the outside of the chest, is not always sufficient to allow the precise problem to be identified. Use of a catheter means that an electrode can be placed inside one of the heart chambers, right up against the heart muscle itself.

Inserting several electrodes into the heart's chambers allows a doctor to chart the progress of an electric current through the muscle. The current may be the one produced by the heart itself. Alternatively, the heart muscle can be deliberately stimulated in a particular way by passing a current into the muscle through one of the implanted electrodes. Either way, the spreading of electrical activity is recorded, revealing where there are obstacles to conduction or where there are short-circuits of the electrical system.

'Contrast' studies to image the heart

The second use of catheters is to allow us to picture the living heart in greater detail than is possible using conventional X-ray techniques. The general problem is that the heart and blood vessels are all made of similar 'soft' material, and so tend to show up as an undifferentiated grey mass on X-ray plates. To reveal its structure we have to introduce some contrast where none exists naturally. This is done by injecting a liquid (called contrast medium) into different parts of the heart. The 'contrast' blocks the passage of X-rays and so shows up white on the X-ray image.

Injecting 'contrast' into an atrium or a ventricle clearly reveals its shape and size. Areas of ventricle that are dead or receiving inadequate oxygen do not contract along with healthier regions of the heart wall. A portion of ventricle will therefore seem to move abnormally, and the outline of the heart chamber will have an odd shape when the muscle contracts. Any weakness in the heart wall that causes it to balloon outwards – a problem called an *aneurysm* – can also be located using contrast studies.

Since blood is travelling through the heart all the time, and the contrast is carried along with it, taking a rapid sequence of X-ray images on film shows how blood is moving. Such film can show, for example, the quantity of blood pumped in a single beat. In the healthy heart, around 70 per cent of the contents of the ventricle is pumped out with each contraction. With heart disease, though, this 'ejection fraction' may be as low as 20 per cent.

Coronary angiography: mapping the coronary arteries

Catheter investigations involving contrast are called angiography.

Among the most useful are studies that outline not the cardiac chambers but the blood vessels – the coronary arteries – that supply the heart muscle. This is *coronary angiography* (see figure 3.2).

Placing a catheter inside a coronary artery is one of the most skilled jobs in medicine. But it is now done routinely, and with very little risk. A recent estimate suggests that the heart develops a serious abnormality of rhythm on one occasion in a hundred, and that the chance of death is around one in five hundred. Coronary angiography is advised for patients who may have serious coronary heart disease. It is often the only way of telling exactly how great the problem is, and establishing whether the patient will best be helped by drugs or by surgical treatment. Coronary angiography is a necessary part of the planning for coronary artery surgery, an operation that significantly improves life expectancy for certain groups of patients. The small risk involved in the investigation is therefore usually considered acceptable.

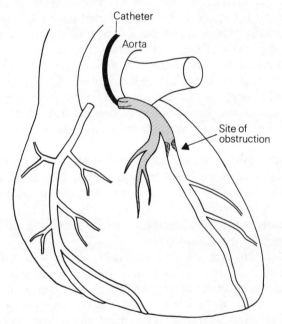

Figure 3.2   Mapping the coronary arteries by coronary angiography. 'Contrast' medium injected by catheter into the opening of the left coronary artery fills its length except where a blockage (arrowed) obstructs the flow of blood. (On normal X-rays contrast appears white because the films are generally viewed as negatives.)

The technique is shown in figure 3.2. The catheter is inched along an artery and down the arch of the aorta, where it is moved right to the base of the blood vessel, immediately above the aortic valve. The catheter tip is then manipulated into one or other of the small holes that mark the start of the two coronary arteries. Contrast injected at this point is swept along the narrow artery, filling the full diameter and length of the vessel. Following the progress of the contrast on X-ray film clearly shows where the blood vessel becomes narrow because of disease or (perhaps) where it is completely blocked. In this way coronary angiography establishes both the severity of any obstruction and its exact position. It is only because of this detailed information that surgery to bypass diseased portions of coronary artery has become possible.

Catheter laboratories

For the measurement of pressures and blood oxygen levels within the heart, it is not necessary to take X-rays during the procedure. But where the passage of contrast is to be tracked through the heart or coronary arteries, there will be sophisticated equipment recording it on cine film or video. Usually X-rays are taken both from the front of the patient and from a little to one side, giving two views of the heart. Though the procedure is complicated, modern equipment allows cardiac catheter studies to be completed in 15–30 minutes. However, if a range of investigations is needed, this period will be longer.

Whereas most diagnostic aids are available in smaller hospitals, 'cath labs' tend to be found in large centres with more specialist medical and technical staff. It is usual for people to spend between one and three days in hospital for catheterisation to be carried out. When contrast is injected for angiography studies some patients feel a hot flush for a few moments.

Development of a new technique called digital subtraction angiography should eventually allow more detailed images to be obtained using smaller amounts of contrast. Another advantage is that the contrast can be injected into an easily accessible vein in the arm (instead of directly into the blood vessel being investigated). Two X-rays are taken, the first before the contrast medium is injected, and the second afterwards. Both images are then converted to digital values by computer. 'Subtracting' the first picture from the second removes most of the background, allowing the feature filled with contrast to stand out more clearly.

Chemicals to track blood and image the heart

One way of studying cardiac performance is to insert a catheter and inject contrast directly into a heart chamber, tracking its progress on X-ray. Another way of following the movement of blood is to introduce into the circulation substances that are slightly radioactive and then to follow them with a camera sensitive to the emission of radioactivity.

This can be done with a single, quick injection of radioactive tracer into a vein. Blood containing the tracer returns to the heart, flows through it to the lungs, back again, and then out to the body. Meanwhile, a machine called a gamma camera (positioned above the patient) 'counts' the amount of radioactivity passing through the different chambers of the heart. Such studies show how much blood is being pumped with each contraction, and the contribution being made by different areas of heart muscle. They are also used to detect abnormal connections between blood vessels and the heart, and holes in the walls between the chambers. Technetium-99 is one of the radioactive substances – known as radio-isotopes – commonly used for this purpose. Another is an isotope of gold.

A variation on the method just described is to take some of a patient's own blood, 'label' the red blood cells with a radioactive chemical, and then re-inject them into a vein. The radioactive tracer becomes mixed throughout the body's blood pool and the gamma camera can then take any number of 'pictures' of the heart, using a computer to ensure each one is synchronised with a particular point in the heart's cycle of contraction and relaxation. The technique is called 'multiple-gated angiography', and the image obtained is commonly referred to as a MUGA scan.

Apart from the initial injection, these procedures, together known as nuclear angiography, are 'non-invasive'. There is no need even for minor surgery, and no equipment has to be placed within the heart. The gamma camera itself is a large saucer-like detector positioned over the chest; but it does not come into contact with the patient.

Any mention of radioactivity is likely to raise eyebrows. However, the kind of radioactivity emitted by radio-isotopes is not dangerous, and the dose to which a patient is exposed is very small: less, for example, than with a normal X-ray. Because of this, radio-isotope scans can be repeated, showing how efficiently the heart works after exercise as well as when the patient is resting. They can also be used to follow the effects of therapy.

The value of isotopes is not confined to measuring heart function. As well as allowing blood to be tracked, technetium has the useful property of becoming concentrated in heart tissue that has died. Dead muscle caused by a heart attack therefore shows up as a bright, 'hot spot' when the gamma camera makes an image of the amount of radioactivity coming from different parts of the heart. Exactly the opposite effect is found when radioactive thallium is injected into the circulation. This substance is absorbed only by heart muscle that has a good supply of blood. So areas that are dead, or supplied by coronary arteries that are narrowed or blocked, show up as dark patches on a gamma camera image.

Other types of scan

A major recent advance in X-ray technology is computerised tomography (CT or 'CAT' scanning, for short). By linking X-ray machines to sophisticated computers, the body can now be 'looked at' from different angles and a series of very precise cross-sectional images built up. The result is something like a series of pictorial 'bacon slices' through the body. So far, the technique has been most useful for parts of the body, like the brain, that do not move. But current developments will allow repeated X-ray images to be taken in time with the heart's rhythm. Movement is therefore frozen at a particular point in the cycle. This development in CT scanning will almost certainly bring significant advance in our ability accurately to diagnose heart disease.

Nuclear magnetic resonance is an entirely different principle of scanning, using magnetic fields and radiofrequency beams to make chemical nuclei in the body's cells behave like tiny radiotransmitters. The potential of this technique is discussed in chapter 11.

Chapter Four

Heart Attack :
What Happens, Why
and What To Do

The heart itself needs fuel: the oxygen and nutrients supplied by blood flowing through the coronary arteries. As with any muscle, the more work the heart has to do, the more fuel it needs. If the demand temporarily outstrips supply (as it may do when someone with coronary artery disease takes exercise, for example), heart muscle protests at the shortage of oxygen. This complaint is made clear to us as the pain of angina (which we return to in chapter 6). When the supply of blood to heart muscle is cut off altogether – as happens when an important coronary artery becomes completely blocked – the muscle dies. In medical terms this process is called *myocardial infarction*; in more familiar language, a heart attack or a 'coronary'.

Generally, the long-term cause of a heart attack is a disease – called *atherosclerosis* – that gradually silts up the coronary arteries. Almost all adults in the Western world have hearts that show signs of this condition, though it is severe enough to cause symptoms only in a minority. Despite its slow development, often beginning around puberty, the most obvious sign of the disease – the heart attack – is a sudden event. Its immediate cause is probably the obstruction of an already narrowed blood vessel by the formation of a blood clot, or thrombus: hence the term coronary thrombosis, which is also used to describe a heart attack. The disease process that underlies the 'furring up' of our arteries, and the immediate events leading to a heart attack are described in the section on coronary artery disease in chapter 2.

Any damage to its muscle threatens to reduce the heart's ability to power the circulation. If the area deprived of oxygen is sufficiently large, the heart starts to pump inefficiently, the circulation begins to fail and life is threatened. Fortunately, the heart is served by a branching network of coronary artery fuel pipes. Usually, at any one time, complete blockage affects only a small part of the whole system (figure 4.1); and for this reason the majority of heart attacks do not cause a failure of the muscular pump itself.

However, damage even to small areas of heart tissue may be critical if the heart's electrical control-system is affected. About 50 per cent of heart attacks are fatal; and around half of these deaths occur within one or two hours of the onset of symptoms. Many

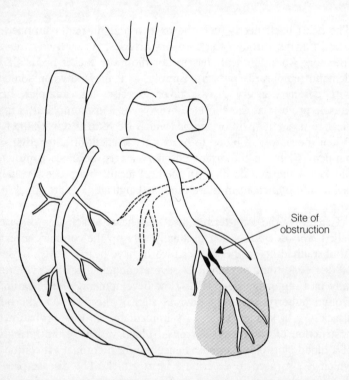

Site of
obstruction

Figure 4.1 Complete blockage of the coronary artery in the place shown will generally lead to death of heart muscle in the shaded area. The terms *heart attack*, *coronary thrombosis*, *a coronary* and the medical description *myocardial infarction* all refer to this event. The area of dead muscle is called an *infarct*.

happen within minutes. The great bulk of these deaths are caused by disturbances in the heart's electrical system.

An abrupt slowing of the heart rate, or complete stoppage, is one form of electrical complication. It occurs when the tracts of tissue that conduct electrical impulses through the heart are damaged. The more usual problem, though, is fast and totally chaotic electrical activity, called *ventricular fibrillation*. Once the heart's electrical signals degenerate to this point, all coordinated pumping action is lost, and death follows within minutes if the condition is not reversed. We do not know why these 'electrical storms' occur during a heart attack.

In Britain, around a quarter of a million people each year have a heart attack. About one in three dies before he or she reaches medical help, mostly because the damaged heart loses its proper rhythm. Not much progress has been made in preventing these deaths since there is so little time to intervene.

In a few years, we may see the wider availability of drugs (such as lignocaine) that reduce the risk of ventricular fibrillation. Ambulance personnel could be allowed to administer them, and people at high risk of heart attack might even have a supply in their own home. (We return to this question in chapter 11). But, for the moment, we are left only with the comforting thought that people who live through the first hour or so of a heart attack have increasingly good chances of long-term survival (figure 4.2). When the heart attack is uncomplicated over the first few hours, the risk of death over the next week is around one in twenty. Improved

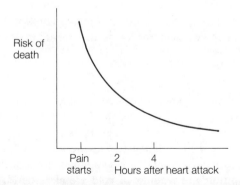

Figure 4.2 Most deaths from heart attack occur in the first few hours.

drug treatment and the possible use of clot-dissolving drugs (also described in chapter 11) should improve the chances still further. Within the next decade we are likely to see something of a revolution in the way heart attacks are handled.

What happens during a heart attack?

Two coronary arteries supply blood to heart muscle, though the left coronary artery divides so quickly that we talk in terms of three major vessels. Each major artery branches, and then branches again until the whole of the cardiac muscle is supplied. Networks of vessels extend not just over the outer surface of the heart but also penetrate the heart muscle throughout its thickness.

The area of heart muscle damaged in a heart attack depends on the exact position of the blockage in the blood supply. Comparison with a tree makes the position clear. Block the progress of sap at a point near the main trunk, and the large area of branches and leaves beyond will wither and die; but if the supply is cut off at one of the smaller branches, less damage is done.

If the blocked blood vessel is small, the area it has to supply is small, and the resulting region of dead muscle – the *infarct* – is small also. The larger the vessel at the point where it is blocked, the greater the amount of heart muscle in danger of dying, and the higher the risk that the heart attack will be fatal, or have severe long-term consequences. Heart muscle that has died does not grow back. Any area affected therefore makes no further contribution to the pumping power of the heart. Another important factor determining the severity of a heart attack is the particular vessel affected, since the coronary arteries differ in the contribution they make to fuelling the left ventricle, which is the most important pumping chamber.

How does someone know they are having a heart attack?

Severe, 'crushing', 'suffocating' chest pain is the major symptom of heart attack. As well as being felt in the centre of the chest, the pain can spread to one or both arms and the neck and jaw. Sweating, nausea, vomiting and feelings of cold are also found; and breathlessness may be experienced. Another frequent feature of a heart attack is something that can only be described as a 'feeling of impending doom'. Pain caused by a heart attack does not vary with breathing or changes in position. It is not relieved by rest.

Some people are absolutely certain they are having a heart attack. But there are many cases where neither patient nor doctor knows for sure. Small areas of heart muscle may die without causing any symptoms, and so are called silent infarcts. Other heart attacks cause only minor disturbances, often passed off at first as 'indigestion'.

Though usually lasting longer, the pain of a heart attack may be similar initially to severe angina, which has the same basic cause. For this reason too, patients sometimes delay seeking assistance. A recent study from the Nottingham area suggests that heart attack patients who eventually call their family doctors wait, on average, three or four hours before doing so. This is far too long. When in any doubt, call for medical help: that is the cardinal rule. Anyone who thinks he or she may be having a heart attack should not delay in the hope that things will improve. A clear account of the type of pain and when it was first felt will help any doctor contacted to decide what action to take.

Coronary arteries narrow enough for a blood clot to cause a sudden heart attack have probably been supplying less blood than the heart needs for many months. The heart, in turn, will have been pumping less efficiently; and the supply of blood to other organs will have been reduced, particularly during exercise. For this reason, a heart attack may be heralded by weeks of tiredness and feeling generally unwell, even though there has been no pain. However, many people who have heart attacks describe the event as totally without warning. Only 25 per cent of people who have a heart attack are known to have had angina or high blood pressure before the event. If someone does have angina, an increase in the frequency of pain may precede the heart attack. But in many cases there is again no warning.

Confirming the heart attack

The symptoms that a patient describes provide good evidence of a heart attack. However, there is little in an initial physical examination that can confirm the diagnosis. People with the characteristic symptoms are therefore treated on the assumption that they have had a heart attack, and the final diagnosis is made later. As we have

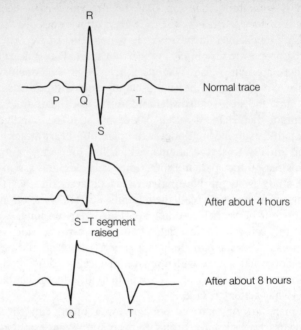

Figure 4.3 ECG changes that may appear in the hours after a heart attack.
The third trace shows a large Q wave; the T wave now appears below the
line instead of above.

said, not all chest pain comes from the heart. This means that
patients may be admitted with suspected heart attack (and have a
couple of days specialised hospital care) when they have not in fact
had one.

Quite often, even the ECG shows none of the classic signs of a
heart attack until several hours after symptoms were first felt. Then
it begins to go through a series of changes which chart the developing damage to heart muscle. The normal ECG pattern is shown
in figure 4.3, together with ECG traces showing the evolution of a
heart attack. These patterns are typical, but they do not always
occur.

Within a few hours, the portion of the ECG trace between the
normal S and T waves starts to rise. Then there develops a pronounced downward deflection of the Q wave; and the T wave,
which normally rises above the line, sinks below it. Though the ST
segment often returns to baseline, and the T wave rights itself, Q

waves usually remain as a permanent sign indicating an area of dead heart muscle. There are characteristic patterns according to the position of the heart muscle affected, and the size of the infarct; but in some patients the ECG remains essentially normal throughout a heart attack.

Along with other muscle, heart cells that are damaged release characteristic chemicals. ECG traces are therefore always interpreted in conjunction with tests that measure the concentration of these enzymes circulating in the patient's blood. Typically, blood samples taken over the first three or so days after a heart attack show a steep rise and then a gradual fall in enzyme levels. Creatine kinase (or CK) is one of the most useful enzymes measured. It reaches a peak 24–48 hours after the heart attack and levels remain raised for three to five days in all. Other enzymes measured include AST (called SGOT in North America) and LDH.

We mentioned in chapter 3 that small quantities of mildly radioactive chemicals are sometimes given to patients as an aid to diagnosis. These chemicals become concentrated in heart muscle that has recently died. Viewing the heart with a gamma camera that measures radioactivity therefore allows doctors to identify more exactly the site and size of infarcts. At the moment, however, few hospitals use this equipment.

Treatment at home or in hospital?

Clearly, the great majority of heart attacks occur outside hospital. Some are so minor that they go almost unnoticed, and may never receive the attention of a doctor. But it is more common for the heart attack to produce severe enough chest pain for a doctor to be called. If someone collapses or is clearly extremely unwell, the result is usually an emergency request for an ambulance. Certain regions in the UK have specialist coronary ambulances which attend cases of suspected heart attack. In effect, these vehicles are mobile coronary care units with specially trained crews; and their ability to treat life-threatening disturbances of heart rhythm probably saves lives. In North America, the system of coronary ambulances and specially trained personnel is well developed. There is now increasing emphasis in Britain on training ambulance staff in the immediate care of patients with heart attack.

It is now usual for people with a heart attack to be admitted to hospital. This will almost certainly happen if an ambulance is summoned, and when the heart attack occurs away from home. However, when the family doctor is called to a patient's house (which often also implies that the start of symptoms has not been dramatic), there may be several good reasons for treating the heart attack without recourse to hospital. If that is a doctor's considered advice, there is no need for alarm.

An average British general practitioner (GP) sees around ten patients each year with heart attack, and is therefore experienced in handling the emergency. When no disturbances of rhythm have developed, and where it seems that the size of the attack is not large enough to threaten the pumping capacity of the heart, a family doctor may suggest that admission to hospital is not necessary. Staying in familiar surroundings reduces the patient's anxiety, and so may lessen the chances that an abnormality of heart rhythm will develop. There is reason to think that older people in particular may be better off if treated at home.

Another important factor is the time between the onset of symptoms and the arrival of the doctor. If four hours or more have passed, the most dangerous period is already over, and the advantage of having easy access to emergency hospital facilities is clearly less. In the recent Nottingham study, a hospital team travelled out to see patients who had initially called their GP. Home treatment was judged appropriate for most of these people. Of those who stayed, only one in ten was later transferred to hospital with complications such as rhythm disturbance and signs of heart failure.

Appendix 6 (and a brief account in the next section) describes what to do if someone collapses with a heart attack. Knowing exactly how to respond can save life in the crucial period before medical help arrives.

Controlling pain and abnormal rhythms

Wherever the heart attack is treated, a doctor has two absolute priorities: to relieve pain and to control the heart if it develops a serious disturbance of rhythm. Doctors will also do whatever possible to reduce the amount of heart muscle damaged, though (as we will see) our ability to intervene in this process is still very limited.

It is said that only someone who has experienced a heart attack knows how grateful a person can be to have pain relieved. Treatment in these circumstances is usually by intravenous injection of drugs from the opiate family of chemicals. Diamorphine (heroin) is often the drug used in Britain. Pain relief is fast and effective; and that alone often improves the condition of the patient's heart. The pain of a heart attack subsides after a few hours, even if untreated, once the heart muscle cells in the affected area have died.

A fast heart rate is a normal response to anxiety and the heart's natural answer to the events of the heart attack itself. A certain irregularity of rhythm is also quite usual. However, if the rate is faster than around 160 beats per minute, the heart's pumping action becomes ineffective. Heart rate and rhythm can often be returned to normal by the injection of drugs which slow the beat and steady irregularities in the pattern of contraction and relaxation. Use of an electric shock can also jolt it into a slower and more efficient rhythm. When the heart beats so chaotically that there is no coordinated rhythm at all – a state called *fibrillation* – the circulation of blood ceases and the brain is deprived of oxygen. Delay of three minutes usually results in permanent brain damage or death. Prompt treatment is therefore essential. The vital requirements are to maintain a circulation (which can be done by repeatedly pressing down on the chest above the heart) and to ensure that oxgyen reaches the blood, using mouth-to-mouth respiration if needed. These basic life support techniques (outlined in appendix 6) should gain enough time for more specific resuscitation to be organised.

Delivery of an electric shock stops the ineffective quivering of heart muscle, and in most cases returns it to a normal rhythm. The device used – the defibrillator – consists of a large battery, with two paddle-shaped electrodes that are placed on the patient's chest. Patients are unconscious and so do not feel the defibrillating shock. Treatment by drugs, given by mouth or directly into a vein, will often reduce the chance that abnormal heart rhythms will recur. Lignocaine, which has already been mentioned, is likely to be one of the first agents used in hospital.

If the infarct affects the heart's electrical conduction system, abnormally slow heart rates can also occur: a condition called *brady-cardia*. Rates of 40 or 50 beats per minute are too low adequately to support the circulation, and need to be speeded up using drugs such as atropine and isoprenaline (given by intravenous injection).

Normal heart rate can also be maintained using a temporary pacemaker. A wire is inserted into a vein and pushed into the right
ventricle of the heart. The delivery of small, regular electric shocks
from an external battery then stimulates its contraction. (Pacemakers
are fully described in chapter 7.)

Doctors are also able to help with other problems that may occur.
Anxiety can be reduced and sleep encouraged by use of diazepam
or a similar tranquilliser; and any nausea and vomiting can be
stopped with drugs. Most important, at home and in hospital, there
is the reassurance that everything possible is being done.

Can heart muscle be saved?

When someone with a heart attack is brought into hospital, there
is a good opportunity for doctors to control unpredictable irregularities of heart rhythm and support the heart through periods when
it threatens to fail. That is the purpose of specialist coronary care
units, which work well in controlling the complications of heart
attack, should any occur. However, even in hospital, there is still
no widely available and agreed way of preventing the death of
heart muscle once the heart attack has occurred. This position will
probably change greatly in the next decade. Chapter 11 covers likely
developments. But for the moment it is sufficient to explain the
problems.

Heart muscle that is completely deprived of blood is dead within
hours. Other muscle in the body is less quickly affected; but the
cells that make up heart tissue cannot switch for long to an internal
chemistry that does not depend on oxygen. Saving the region of
muscle that is supplied exclusively by the blocked artery therefore
requires immediate action. Even if we knew what to do we could
probably not do it in time.

However, around the area of heart muscle that has no blood is a
larger region in which the supply has been reduced but not completely cut off. This muscle is threatened, but could perhaps be
saved, if the *supply* of blood to the border zone were increased or
its *demand* for oxygen reduced. Many drugs have been tried with
the aim of lessening the area of ultimate damage. They include
beta-blockers and calcium antagonists, which might be expected to
reduce the heart muscle's need for oxygen by slowing heart rate
and decreasing blood pressure. There is recent evidence that giving
beta-blockers immediately after a heart attack reduces the likelihood

of complications (including death) over the first week, even though they do not decrease infarct size. However, other drugs have seemed promising before, and it is too early to say whether this hope will be fulfilled. (Chapter 13 describes these and other drugs used in the treatment of heart disease.) More exotic agents, such as snake venom (which in fact just reduces blood clotting), have also been tried. But none so far has been widely accepted as effective. Efforts to restore the flow of blood seem, at the moment, to be more promising. Drugs such as streptokinase have the potential to dissolve clots and are under trial. There are also mechanical means of re-opening blocked coronary arteries. The technique of angioplasty, in which a tiny balloon is inflated inside the blood vessel to squeeze the sides apart, is one of them. In the USA, emergency surgery to bypass the obstructed coronary artery is also increasingly used. Coronary artery bypass is a routine treatment for angina, and is described in chapter 6. Other developments are considered in chapter 11.

However, until these methods are perfected, hospital treatment for most patients is confined to preventing complications, and providing support for the heart and circulation. This is usually done in coronary care units or in other specialist wards. A feature of these wards is the intensive monitoring of patients. (Many people with heart attacks are in fact looked after in general intensive care units that also deal with other seriously ill patients.) Numerous machines check vital functions and sound alarms should anything go wrong. Particularly noticeable are the oscilloscope screens on which patients' ECG traces are continuously displayed.

Here and back on the general ward, the aim is to provide the best environment in which the heart can heal itself. Shortly after the heart attack, muscle around the central area of dying tissue starts to swell. This further reduces the flow of blood and enlarges the infarct. But then healing proper begins. Though heart muscle never regrows, cells infiltrate the area, scavenging away dead material and replacing it with interlacing fibres that eventually form a firm scar.

Why are some heart attacks more serious than others?

We mentioned earlier that the severity of a heart attack depends on the size of the muscle area deprived of oxygen, and also on the *site* of the infarct. Clearly certain areas of muscle are particularly important.

If there is an infarct in the muscle wall between the heart's beating chambers, the result may be a hole that allows blood to short-circuit its proper route through the lungs. If muscle anchoring the flaps of one of the heart valves is affected, the valve may start to leak, even though a similarly small area of dead muscle elsewhere in the heart may hardly be noticed. Clearly, there are also vital areas of muscle where any infarction will interrupt the system of electrical conduction, and so compromise heart rate and rhythm.

Though one blood vessel is completely shut off, it remains possible that blood may reach the threatened heart muscle by a roundabout route. The severity of a heart attack therefore also depends on whether there is any 'collateral circulation'. Gradual narrowing of the coronary arteries over many years allows time for blood vessels to grow around the developing obstruction. This means that even if the main channel is blocked, enough blood gets through along side routes for the muscle to survive. For this reason, a small heart attack in a young man (whose heart has previously been healthy) may do more damage than the same-sized attack in an older man whose disease has been slow in developing and whose coronary circulation has therefore had time to adapt.

Finally, there is the fact that damage to the heart muscle is cumulative, since an area of tissue that dies does not regrow. This means that a series of small infarctions – the earlier ones being hardly noticed – may ultimately undermine the pumping efficiency of the heart as completely as a single large heart attack.

Other problems that may follow a heart attack

Heart failure

Many people entering hospital after a heart attack show mild and temporary signs of heart failure. This sounds a dangerous condition, but can usually be reversed with reasonably simple drug treatment. A heart that is pumping less efficiently sends less blood through the kidneys, and the patient produces little urine. The volume of blood therefore increases, placing additional strain on the heart and leading to the waterlogging of tissues, including the lungs. This build-up of fluid can produce breathlessness. It may also be apparent as crackling noises in the lungs that can be heard with a stethoscope, and can often be seen on a chest X-ray. The first line of drug therapy is with agents called diuretics that increase urine flow and so reduce the volume of circulating blood and the strain on the heart.

Where dealing with the problem would be made easier by knowing exactly how much blood the heart is pumping, it may be useful to measure the performance of the heart directly. Such techniques are described towards the end of chapter 3. Steps taken to support the patient at risk of serious heart failure involve complicated drug regimes and the insertion into the heart of instruments that monitor its function.

Embolism

Patients who spend long periods in bed are at risk of developing blood clots in their leg veins, where blood moves relatively slowly. (The condition is called deep vein thrombosis.) There is a danger that these clots may travel through the circulation to the right side of the heart and from there into the lungs, where they become lodged. This is called *pulmonary embolism*. Small vessels blocked in this way can give rise to breathlessness and infections; if large vessels are blocked, the clot may be fatal.

Blood clots can also form on areas of damaged muscle within the left side of the heart. These clots occasionally break free and travel through the body's arteries until they become lodged in organs such as the brain, where they cause stroke.

The problem of embolism is tackled in two ways: by encouraging patients to be out of bed and active as soon as the condition of their heart permits; and by giving anti-coagulant drugs that 'thin the blood' and so reduce its tendency to clot. Anti-coagulant drugs are particularly valuable in patients who have had previous problems with embolism and so are known to be at risk.

Aneurysms and surgical repair of the heart

Though tough scar tissue usually replaces dead muscle, the heart wall may become thin where the infarct took place. When the ventricle contracts, the wall can bulge at this point, absorbing part of the energy of the heart's contraction and contributing to its poor performance. This balloon-like abnormality of the heart wall is called an *aneurysm*. Surgery to remove it may help the heart beat more efficiently.

Other damage to the structure of the heart may be serious enough to require surgery: to repair holes in the beating chambers or replace damaged valves. It is best that such problems are recognised and dealt with early, before the heart begins to fail and survival is threatened by its effect on other organs. Certain of these problems can be controlled by drugs, but many require prompt surgery. Although the risk of operating soon after a heart attack is high, it is better to correct these defects before the patient's condition deteriorates any further.

Chapter Five

After a Heart Attack : Returning to a Full Life

With every day that passes after a heart attack, the chances of a severe complication decrease. For this reason, the majority of patients, who do not develop any particular problems, are able to leave the specialised coronary care unit within two to three days of their arrival, and will probably be discharged from hospital in a week or ten days. Over this initial period of recovery, there is a substantial increase in the amount of physical activity that can be regarded as safe. Most people feel well enough to sit up in bed once the initial pain has been controlled, and begin to walk around the ward in a day or two. After a week they will probably be as mobile as anyone in the hospital, and can then think seriously about going home. These are only very broad generalisations, however. Every patient is different, and every doctor too. Advice in any individual case can therefore vary a great deal, without implying that anything is wrong; and some doctors prefer a more cautious approach during the early days after a heart attack.

Attitudes, beliefs and personality affect response to illness, including heart disease, and influence a person's chances of survival and physical recovery. They also play a vital part in determining quality of life. Except in those few people whose hearts have been very severely affected, the amount of disability that follows a heart attack seems to depend as much on attitudes to the illness, and on personality, social circumstances and family relationships, as it does on the state of the heart itself. Evidence from a recent, large study in West Germany suggests that the longer heart attack patients stay in bed and in hospital, the more anxious and pessimistic they become. The aim is therefore to return to normal – or better than normal – as quickly as possible. No-one should regard themselves as a 'heart case' just because they have had a heart attack.

Coming to terms

Nevertheless, having a heart attack is undeniably a frightening, life-threatening and initially painful experience. It is a crisis which may provoke profound psychological reactions, both at the time of the attack and in the months that follow. 'Why me?' is a common question. It is asked with particular feeling by previously fit people who have prided themselves on being physically active. The answer is that not everyone with a healthy lifestyle can avoid heart disease, just as not everyone with unhealthy pastimes suffers from it. Many of the factors responsible for heart attacks lie in our individual genetic make-up, and so cannot be altered. Others are probably environmental influences of which we are not yet aware. Decisions that we make may increase or decrease the chances of heart disease (*see* chapter 12); but there is no certainty, and little point after the event in trying to lay blame.

Along with attempts to find fault, depression, irritability and fear (of death and of the end of an established pattern of life) are common and entirely understandable responses. Minor tranquilliser and anti-depressant drugs for short periods can bring effective relief; so too can the opportunity to talk with others who are undergoing similar problems. But the most useful help is probably *understanding* – of what has happened and what the future may hold.

When people who have had heart attacks discuss their fears and feelings, several common problems emerge. One immediate difficulty is in adjusting to life outside the coronary care unit (CCU). In the CCU, a patient is constantly monitored by equipment and watched over by nursing staff. It feels safe. On a general ward, supervision is far less intense. Initial insecurity is therefore a natural reaction. There is a similar feeling of vulnerability when someone leaves hospital altogether. Some patients express it by making sure their daily walks take them near the hospital, or by continuing to wear their hospital identity bracelets.

Both in the move from the CCU and in leaving hospital, it is important to remember that the level of medical watchfulness relates directly to the chance of there being a serious complication. After a couple of days, there is little likelihood that anything will go seriously wrong, and less again with each passing day.

Feelings of disorientation and insecurity may be less marked if a heart attack is treated by a doctor at home, where illness is more easily integrated into daily life. The person affected does not have to cope with such radical changes in role: first becoming a hospital patient, highly dependent on others even for the most basic and intimate care; and then once more assuming autonomy.

When someone has been in hospital, the return to spouse and family may be as difficult for those at home as for the patient. A recent study of male patients from King's College Hospital in London identified several sources of problems. Many of the men's wives were unconcerned once the heart attack had been dealt with in hospital, and optimistic about the future. However, others felt guilty of causing their husbands' illness; or were angry at their husbands for having brought the problem on themselves by self-neglect: smoking too much, perhaps, or overwork. Most felt a special responsibility for overseeing their husbands' rehabilitation, and some anticipated difficulty in persuading their spouses to keep to medical advice. Particularly if they are left unexpressed, any of these feelings can become a source of friction, and contribute to depression and anxiety.

On the part of the men, return home brought a sense of isolation, since many felt unable to discuss problems freely with their families. In some cases this was because the family needed them to appear strong, even when they were not. In others, ex-patients were afraid to acknowledge difficulties because they felt their families wanted to label them as invalids, and treat them as such. Someone who has had a heart attack needs to be able to admit to anxiety without it being seized upon as an example of weakness.

The point that comes out most clearly from the King's College Hospital study, and from many other studies of heart attack, is that the patient's spouse and close family are strongly affected. They have to cope with the practical difficulties of sudden illness; but also with its emotional consequences, which seem to be as severe for them as for the patient. On the negative side, there is a suggestion that many families are inclined to be overprotective, and that this can delay recovery. More positively, families provide the most important source of support. Many hospitals are therefore beginning to involve patients' wives and husbands in rehabilitation, having them along to discussions between patient and doctor, and encouraging their participation in self-help groups. Nevertheless, spouses still often complain that they have not been sufficiently involved, nor given enough information.

However it is dealt with, it is not surprising that having a heart attack often brings some degree of change. The illness itself may produce poor concentration and fatigue, which persists for a time and restricts activities. Though most people of working age return to their jobs, often after four to six weeks, it is usual to be working rather less hard even a year after the heart attack. There is a similar small decrease, on average, in leisure activities. Social contact and sexual activity are rated as unchanged by one patient in two; some experience a slight increase (one in five patients says that his or her marriage has improved), but others suffer a substantial decrease. (Misunderstandings about the risks involved in having sex after a heart attack are considered in the next section.)

Change may be resisted, grudgingly accepted as inevitable or actively seized upon as an opportunity to improve one's quality of life. Recovery from illness is a chance to take stock: to review the past, and decide how life should proceed from here. For some, this might mean taking extra holidays, pursuing a long-neglected hobby, retiring to the country or spending more time with the family. For many, the result is an enrichment of life rather than its limitation.

Exercise

Not long ago, patients with a heart attack were in bed for three weeks (the first spent lying flat on their backs) and in hospital for six. Medical views have changed much over the past 20 years, and doctors are now far more encouraging about a quick return to a physically active life. Tests which monitor the ECG while a person exercises contribute to the view that progressive increases in activity can safely be encouraged in the majority of patients, who should be started on the road to physical recovery while they are still in the coronary care unit. The exercise test (described in chapter 3) also gives valuable self-confidence to the patient, showing levels of exercise that can be achieved without the appearance of abnormal changes in the heart.

People who have left hospital will probably not want to be confined to their beds. In the first few days at home, it is good to be up, dressed, and possibly out in the garden (though taking early nights and naps if tired is sensible). In the second week, short walks are appropriate. These should increase gradually in length unless chest pain or breathlessness develops, in which case a doctor should be told. As we have mentioned, the heart takes time to heal after an infarct. Over these weeks a scar is slowly forming at the site where the heart was damaged. After a month at home, many patients are happily walking a mile on most days.

Walking is a rhythmic activity that uses the body's major groups of muscles. So too do swimming and jogging. (People who have recovered from heart attacks have successfully completed marathon races.) All three forms of exercise encourage fitness: a state in which the muscles make increasingly efficient use of oxygen and so reduce demands on the heart. Becoming physically fit should also increase psychological well-being. But there is no point pushing fitness beyond the point at which the activity itself is pleasurable; and explosive forms of exercise, such as squash, place great strain on the heart and ought to be avoided. Jobs involving heavy manual labour should be returned to gradually, perhaps on a part-time basis at first, and with emphasis on less strenuous aspects of the work.

Sex

Advice on their sex life is something heart patients want most and get least of, or so surveys suggest. The basic message is that people should take things easy, but resume sexual relations when they feel like it. As a very general guide, most patients – if they wish – can safely return to sexual activity within a month of a coronary. Doing only what is comfortable for both partners, confidence will gradually return. Lack of interest in sex is normal in the immediate aftermath of a heart attack, when the main concern is for survival, and depression and fatigue are frequent. However, American research suggests that the majority of patients are sexually active again by three months.

Despite popular misconceptions, sex involves no more physical effort than climbing one or two flights of stairs; and the body's response to it is the same as to any exercise. Twenty-four hour ECG recordings in patients show a maximum heart rate of around 120 beats per minute during intercourse. This is no higher than achieved at other points during the day and soon falls to usual levels. So it is wrong to think that returning to the previous pattern of sexual activity poses any special threat to the heart. Evidence for this comes from Japanese researchers who analysed the post-mortem records of more than 5,000 men who died suddenly. Only 34 of these deaths occurred during intercourse.

There is some suggestion that sex with an unaccustomed partner involves greater increases in heart rate and blood pressure, and so might be slightly more risky from the heart's point of view. The Japanese study bears this out. It was found that all but four of the 30 deaths occurred in people who were with a partner other than their spouse. These partners, on average, were also 18 years younger; and there was good evidence that alcohol as well as extra-marital sex had a hand in the outcome. The moral of the story seems to be that heart attacks and sudden death do occur during sexual intercourse, but are extremely rare events within a stable relationship.

People who have angina after a heart attack may find that sex brings on the pain. Warming the bed sheets, not making love after a heavy meal or a hot bath, and taking a nitrate tablet (*see* chapter 6) before intercourse may help. The position adopted during inter-course seems to make little difference to the work of the heart.

Angina is a complication that can affect sex life. So too can any remaining signs of heart failure. In both cases, drugs used to treat the condition may contribute to the difficulty. However, there is a range of drugs that can be used, and it should be possible to find a treatment that has little effect on potency or libido. In the absence of particular complications, the size of the heart attack itself seems not to affect the chances of resuming a satisfying sex life.

Driving

The possibility that someone may have a heart attack while driving obviously represents a danger to that person and to others. In practice, most people who are about to have a heart attack seem to have sufficient warning to stop or at least slow down; and heart attacks account for only around 15 per cent of all accidents caused by sudden illness.

In the weeks after a heart attack, the risk of a second coronary or the sudden and serious development of abnormal heart rhythm is not great. Nevertheless, the danger is real, and in Britain people who have had a heart attack must not resume driving within two months of the event. At some time during this period, they should inform the Driver and Vehicle Licensing Centre (Swansea) that they have had a heart attack. Their insurance company should also be told.

After two months, people who have had a heart attack are usually allowed to resume car driving. One exception to this is when angina is easily provoked either by the exertion or emotion of driving. Drivers of heavy goods and public service vehicles (including taxis) are subject to stricter and far more detailed controls. More information about heart disease and driving is given in appendix 3.

Flying – as a passenger – is not likely to be a problem once someone has recovered from the heart attack itself. On the other hand, piloting an aeroplane, either as an amateur or professional, is permitted only under certain stringent conditions.

What are the long-term chances?

The simple answer is 'good'. It would be foolish to deny that someone who has had a heart attack is not at risk of having another. The first heart attack shows that disease is present in the coronary arteries, and this disease cannot be eliminated, though we can take important steps to stop it progressing. But the chances of another heart attack are not great, and they decrease with time. In the first year, there is roughly a one in ten chance of another coronary. In the second year, the risk is down to one in twenty; and after two or three years someone who has had a heart attack is little more likely to suffer one than any other man or woman of the same age.

These are, of course, very general figures. Among certain groups of patients, the outlook is better than this; among others, not as good. For young people with small infarcts, for example, the risk of death in the year following a heart attack is only one in fifty. This is also true of patients whose left ventricles are known to be functioning normally, and when there is no evidence from an exercise test that heart muscle is being deprived of blood. Anyone who has had a heart attack may experience odd twinges of chest pain over a few days or weeks. These are unlikely to be a problem. A minority of people develop a more severe form of chest pain which accompanies exercise or emotion, but then disappears. This is angina, caused by a temporary inability of the coronary arteries to supply the heart muscle with the increased oxygen supply it needs. The next chapter is a detailed description of angina and the options for treatment.

In another small group of patients, the heart's pumping capacity may have been sufficiently damaged for there to be continuing problems of breathlessness and ankle swelling. Repeated heart attacks also lead to signs of heart failure by progressively reducing the ability of the left ventricle to drive the circulation. As with angina, treatment with drugs (*see* chapters 9 and 13) is usually effective in controlling symptoms. However, the outlook for a patient whose heart has been seriously weakened is less good than for those whose infarction was uncomplicated.

Preventing another heart attack

Some people feel that there was nothing they could do to prevent their first heart attack, and that once recovered they are on a one-way road to the next one. The statistics mentioned show that for the average patient this is certainly not the case. For those judged to be at highest risk, there is much that can be done to improve the odds. No heart attack is inevitable. In certain circumstances, medical and surgical treatment will greatly improve the prospects. In others, the answer lies as much in a person's own hands as in those of the doctor.

Anyone who smokes must stop. This is by far the most important message to anyone interested in preventing a heart attack, whether they have had one already or not. Stopping smoking will also help prevent other diseases, such as bronchitis and lung cancer.

Next to that, anyone overweight should try to lose some of the excess. This will reduce strain on the heart, decrease any tendency to angina and help lower blood pressure. Modest exercise with a doctor's advice will help with weight control, but reducing weight will almost certainly involve eating less, or rather eating less of the most fattening foods, notably sugar and fat itself. Alcohol also contributes many superfluous calories. Drinking less therefore makes weight control easier.

For people whose bodies are found to metabolise fats abnormally, strict control of diet may be needed. Such patients are often young, and at high risk of further heart disease (*see* appendix 2 on inheriting high cholesterol). There may also be a case for long-term use of drugs that reduce levels of cholesterol circulating in the blood.

However, for people whose bodies handle fats normally, diet is not something to become obsessive about, apart from any need to lose weight. The argument over the role of dietary cholesterol in heart disease is long and many-sided. Cutting down on dairy products and animal fat, while replacing them with certain kinds of vegetable oil and fish, will do no harm – and may be of benefit. But the issue is not as straightforward as is sometimes suggested. Chapter 12 presents the arguments.

Whether people with stressful jobs should take things easy is another difficult question. Stress may be a cause of heart disease, or simply a factor that precipitates it. We know that stress increases levels of the 'fight and flight' hormones that stimulate the heart and so increase its demand for oxygen; but proving that this short-term effect translates into increased long-term risk is not easy. For someone whose life would seem empty if they stopped work or took a back seat, there is probably no compelling reason to change. But for someone who has decided that high-powered employment is a chore, and would rather be tending grandchildren or the roses, a heart attack may provide the looked-for opportunity to slow down.

Finally, anyone who has had one heart attack is in a good position to deal with another, if they are unlucky enough to suffer a second time. Should the symptoms recur, call quickly for help – either from the family doctor or from the hospital direct. Anyone who has had a heart attack might find it useful to discuss in advance with their General Practitioner which course of action is better.

Can drugs help prevent a second coronary?

We can be reasonably sure that certain drugs reduce the risk of a second heart attack. But whether, on balance, it is worthwhile taking them is still an unresolved question.

One possibility is long-term treatment with drugs called beta-blockers (*see* chapter 13). Over half a dozen studies (involving more than 20,000 patients) have looked at whether such therapy decreases the risk of death from another heart attack over the next 12 months. Considering all their results together, the balance of evidence suggests that taking beta-blockers each day for a year does reduce the risk by a statistically significant – but rather small – amount.

Of the people who survive an initial heart attack, perhaps eight in every 100 die during the following year. If all 100 of these ex-patients take beta blockers throughout the year, we would expect only five or six to die. That is, we would save two to three lives out of eight, a reduction in mortality of between a quarter and a third. This sounds worthwhile enough. But consider the odds another way. For the two or three lives we save in a year, 97 people have to take drugs every day without receiving any benefit: five die despite the extra treatment, and 92 would have survived anyway. Since all drugs have some potential side-effects, the benefit of taking beta-blockers may not be considered justifiable.

This is especially so if we consider different types of patient. Those at greatest risk of another heart attack are people who have had some form of heart failure. Such patients would not be pre-scribed beta-blockers because of the drugs' known tendency to worsen the condition. Beta-blockers would not adversely affect the hearts of young people with small infarcts, but these patients have the lowest risk anyway. They are also the patients most likely to be worried by other drug side-effects such as impotence and restrictions on the ability to exercise.

Having said that, there are reasons for taking a beta-blocker which are not directly to do with the fact that someone has had a heart attack. In people with high blood pressure, beta-blockers have a beneficial effect, reducing the risk of stroke. The drugs are also valuable in preventing angina. So there will be many people who were taking a beta-blocker before their heart attack and who con-tinue to take it afterwards. There will be others who are rec-ommended to start taking the drug only after their heart attack, perhaps because their high blood pressure had not been diagnosed before or perhaps because they have only recently developed angina.

For one reason or another, around a quarter of heart attack patients may be taking a beta-blocker when they leave hospital. However, in those who have no blood pressure problem and no angina, the benefit of blanket prescription of beta-blockers is argu-able. It may be worth trying the drugs; but if side-effects occur, they can be discontinued without fear that anyone is giving up a treatment of major value.

Earlier, we described the immediate cause of heart attack as the formation of a clot, or thrombus, that blocks a narrowed coronary artery. Drugs that might prevent this happening are therefore a logical treatment to try in the attempt to prevent recurrence of the problem.

Clotting involves several processes. One is the formation of an insoluble web of protein strands (made of fibrin), which coagulate blood in the familiar way we see when we cut ourselves. This tends to happen where blood is slow-moving. Clotting also involves the clumping together of blood cell fragments known as platelets. Clots are therefore a mixture of fibrin and platelets.

A few years ago, patients who suffered a heart attack may have been given drugs, such as warfarin, to reduce coagulation. Anti-coagulant drugs are useful where blood flows slowly, but the evidence that they prevent heart attacks is now thought unconvincing. Such drugs also have a distinct disadvantage, since their use may lead to uncontrolled bleeding.

Anti-platelet drugs reduce platelet 'stickiness' and so their tendency to form plugs where blood flows over uneven surfaces. Recently, their use in the prevention of heart attacks has begun to seem more promising.

One common anti-platelet drug is aspirin, though it should be emphasised that the dose needed to affect platelets is far lower than the amount taken to relieve pain. (A junior aspirin every other day gives an idea of the quantity of drug involved.) Evidence obtained by pooling the results of many different trials (each of which was inconclusive on its own) has begun to show measurable benefit: it looks as if aspirin may reduce the risk of a second heart attack by around 20 per cent.

As with beta-blockers, the overall effect of anti-platelet drugs is therefore relatively small. When seen against a background that is already good, it has been difficult to show convincingly that their use is beneficial. However, the low incidence of side-effects with aspirin makes a 'take it just to be on the safe side' policy more justifiable than with beta-blockers. Aspirin after the first heart attack is not routine. But it may be given to certain patients (perhaps those who are particularly young or who have had several coronaries) for two to three years. Other drugs that reduce platelet stickiness are dipyridamole and sulphinpyrazone. Taking them together with aspirin, or with beta-blockers, may bring additional benefit; but the worth of such drug combinations has still to be firmly established.

Chapter Six

Angina

Angina is a problem of supply and demand: an area of heart muscle temporarily requires more blood than the coronary artery serving it is able to provide. The result is pain or discomfort. Since the heart muscle's need for blood varies, depending on the amount of work the heart has to do, angina comes and goes. Often, attacks of pain are brought on by exercise or emotion. The angina disappears once the demand for extra blood has eased, only to return when the workload of the heart is again increased. Unlike the pain of a heart attack, the chest pain of angina is therefore recurrent and short-lived. The heart's coronary arteries may become temporarily constricted because of spasm, when the artery walls contract and so clamp the vessel shut. However, by far the most common cause of angina is a gradual accumulation of fatty deposits – called *atheroma* – along the blood vessel walls. (The way atheroma develops is described in chapter 2.)

So, angina is a *symptom* of coronary artery disease; it is not a disease itself. Doctors treating it are faced with two tasks. The first is to control the pain, so that someone with angina can continue to lead a full life. The second, is to try to prevent the underlying disease developing to the stage when the narrowed coronary artery becomes completely blocked – causing a heart attack, which may impair the pumping ability of the heart and perhaps prove fatal.

Angina affects about two people in every 100 aged between 35 and 60. In this age group, the condition is more than twice as frequent among men as among women. Smokers are twice as likely to suffer as non-smokers.

The severity and frequency of angina vary greatly from one person to another: from occasional mild discomfort to an intense pain, possibly accompanied by feelings of anxiety and suffocation. (The word 'angina' comes from the Greek meaning 'to choke' and has the same root as the terms 'anxiety' and 'anguish'.) At its worst, untreated angina greatly restricts working life and limits social and leisure activities. Fortunately, we now have safe and effective treatments – both medical and surgical – for the condition.

Even so, the diagnosis of angina is worrying – to the person affected and the family. An important part of coming to terms with angina is understanding how the problem arises, and what the symptom means. Such understanding will also help in making decisions when there is a choice between different forms of therapy.

The symptoms

Usually, angina occurs only when the workload on the heart is increased. Typically, angina appears during exercise. The body's muscles demand extra supplies of oxygen and nutrients, requiring an increase in the frequency and force with which the heart pumps blood. Since the heart muscle too is having to work harder, it also needs more fuel. Healthy coronary arteries are able to meet this additional demand with increased flow of blood. However, when they are narrowed by disease, the demand for blood temporarily outstrips their ability to supply it. The heart protests, and pain is experienced.

Angina is felt most often in the region over the breastbone, but it may spread around the chest, and even affect the neck and jaw, shoulders and arms. It is a continuous rather than stabbing pain (sometimes thought of more as an ache), and is frequently described as oppressive, crushing or numbing. Feelings of cold, sweating and breathlessness may accompany the pain.

Severe angina is difficult to distinguish from the symptoms of a heart attack. Indeed, the cause of the pain – lack of oxygen supply to the heart muscle (a condition called *ischaemia*) – is exactly the same. However, there are two important differences in the way the pain occurs. One is that angina is *reversible*. Rest reduces the demand for oxygen to a level which the narrowed coronary artery can satisfy, and so relieves the pain. Angina therefore usually lasts for minutes rather than hours.

The other important point about angina attacks is that they are *predictable*. They tend to occur after a certain amount of physical effort, such as walking uphill or climbing a particular flight of stairs (especially after a heavy meal), and then disappear. As well as exercise (including sex), eating, smoking and emotions such as anger, excitement and fear sometimes precipitate an attack. There may also be a regular association between angina and cold and windy weather.

Putting these two factors together gives us a rough guide. Short-lived and predictable chest pain of the kind described is likely to be angina. But when a severe chest pain lasts ten minutes or longer, has not been experienced before and is not relieved by rest, heart attack is a possibility.

Angina pains and those of a heart attack appear in many guises, and pains similar to those described may be due to problems completely unrelated to the heart. Inflammation of the lining of the lungs (pleurisy) causes chest pain; so too do problems with the oesophagus, which passes just behind the heart. However, all chest pain should be taken seriously; and if it is at all likely that someone is having a heart attack, medical help should be summoned immediately.

The problem of angina may make a gradual appearance, or start to affect someone quite suddenly. The way the condition develops is also unpredictable: it can remain stable for years, or progress in a matter of months from mild pain on strenuous exertion to severe pain with hardly any exercise. Any significant *change* in the pattern of symptoms should be taken as a warning sign. When angina that has been predictable for long periods suddenly starts to appear after far less exertion, or in unexpected circumstances, it is important to obtain medical advice.

We have said that angina is almost always associated with an increase in the heart's workload. However, there can be a progressive worsening of angina symptoms when pain is experienced even though someone is resting, and perhaps asleep. This is often referred to as *unstable angina* and is a serious condition, since there is a clear risk of a heart attack developing. Treatment with drugs that reduce the tendency of the blood to clot (*see* chapter 5) or prompt surgery (described at the end of this chapter) may be recommended.

With the far more common form of angina, associated with exercise, the intensity of angina pain does not necessarily relate to the seriousness of the disease causing it. Extreme narrowing of the coronary arteries may produce only mild pain, or no angina at all;

while many people whose pain is crippling have less severe disease. This means the doctor may suggest a series of steps to find out exactly how seriously the heart is affected.

Investigating angina

Exercise 'stress' tests

Heart muscle receiving insufficient oxygen produces a characteristic pattern of electrical activity. We can therefore obtain useful information from a test called the *exercise ECG* or 'stress test', in which changes in the electrical activity of the heart are recorded as the patient gradually increases the intensity of exercise. Properly interpreted, the test provides important information about the amount of heart muscle that is obtaining insufficient blood, and where that ischaemic muscle is situated.

The exercise test is not much different from an ordinary ECG (EKG), except that the patient is active rather than resting. The activity takes the form of walking on a 'treadmill', a moving belt that gradually increases speed and tilts upwards to simulate walking uphill. To standardise conditions, patients are asked not to eat or take any drugs in the few hours before the test is performed. Further details of the exercise test are given in chapter 3.

The stress test is non-invasive: nothing is inserted into the body, and there is no need for injections. Though the investigation is safe, the exertion involved is sometimes sufficient to bring on the angina pain, in which case the ECG pattern that accompanies its onset may provide particularly valuable evidence about the underlying problem. However, the exercise ECG does not have to induce pain to be useful; and in many patients there is a 'positive' finding on the exercise ECG – indicating insufficient oxygen supply to an area of muscle – even though there is no angina. When there are no ECG changes characteristic of oxygen deficiency the result of the test is described as negative. A negative exercise test is good evidence that there are no serious problems with the coronary arteries.

Making a record of the ECG over 24 hours may be another useful aid to diagnosis in some patients, since the occurrence of pain and of episodes of oxygen deprivation in the heart can be related to the normal lifestyle. Such recordings are made using a simple battery-operated device.

Coronary angiography

We know from the angina pain itself that the heart's blood supply is being restricted at some point in the network of coronary arteries. The pattern of symptoms itself may be all that is needed to decide on the best course of treatment. A great many patients have their angina perfectly well controlled by rest and drugs, and require no further investigations. When it is decided that further information is needed, the exercise ECG gives us more insight into the nature of the problem. But we may still need to establish exactly *where* in the coronary circulation any obstruction lies, and identify the precise *extent* to which the coronary arteries have become narrowed by disease. To help in making the best decisions about treatment, it is often also useful to know whether the pumping performance of the heart has already been damaged by the inadequacy of its blood supply. Putting in place these pieces of the jigsaw requires a short stay in hospital.

Establishing the precise site of any narrowing in the heart's arteries involves a procedure known as *coronary angiography*. A fine tube (called a catheter) is inserted into an arm or leg artery and gently pushed along the blood vessel until it reaches the heart. Fluid that shows up on X-rays is then injected directly into a coronary artery and its progress along the blood vessel followed in a series of exposures. In this way, narrowed portions of coronary artery are revealed. The technique is described in more detail in chapter 3.

Similar procedures can be used to find out how well the left ventricle is working. X-ray contrast fluids injected into the heart are tracked as they pass through the heart chambers, showing how efficiently blood is being pumped. There are also ways of obtaining this information using various forms of heart scan, some of them involving the injection of mildly radioactive chemicals. The advantage of such scans is that they avoid the need to pass catheters into the heart. Chapter 3 again contains more information on these techniques.

Choices in treatment: rest, drugs and surgery

Given that angina is basically a problem of supply and demand, there are two fundamental ways of tackling it. One is to reduce the heart muscle's requirement for blood; the other, to increase its supply. The simplest way of decreasing the demand for blood is to rest. Less exercise means less strain on the heart. When angina occurs only with the most strenuous exercise, avoiding activities that bring on the pain is a practical solution. However, at its most serious, angina is a persistent problem even when there is little exertion. Leading a full life requires that we are active, even if that means no more than being able to climb stairs or walk to the car. Simply 'taking things easy' is therefore only a partial, and often temporary, measure.

The past two decades have brought a variety of effective drugs for controlling angina. The most recent drugs also seem to reduce the risk of a heart attack in certain forms of the disease. Also over the past 20 years, surgeons have developed an operation in which narrowed sections of coronary artery are bypassed by the construction of new blood vessels. This directly restores a good blood supply to affected areas of the heart and so prevents pain that cannot be controlled by drugs. In people with certain patterns of coronary artery disease, surgery also reduces the risk of a heart attack and prolongs life. The range of options available means that patients and their doctors now have considerable choice and can tailor treatment to fit individual circumstances. Deciding on the best course of action is not always straightforward; and doctors, even with the patient's best interests always in mind, may give different advice.

Whatever they recommend, two points are always borne in mind. The first relates to quality of life: the treatment offered should prevent pain and allow the person to enjoy life to the full. Secondly, treatment should prolong life. Angina is a symptom of coronary artery disease, the other face of which is a heart attack. The presence of angina is a warning that the system of coronary arteries is being progressively obstructed. When these obstructions occur at certain critical points, there is an appreciable threat to life. Treating angina therefore involves complicated decisions relating to diagnosis and treatment. Typically, the process of decision-making involves a series of steps similar to those outlined in figure 6.1.

A patient with angina-like chest pain will probably first consult his family doctor. Where the condition is thought to be mild, this may be sufficient. Treatment will usually involve rest, and probably drugs to prevent or relieve the pain. However, if there is any suspicion of serious underlying disease, the patient will probably

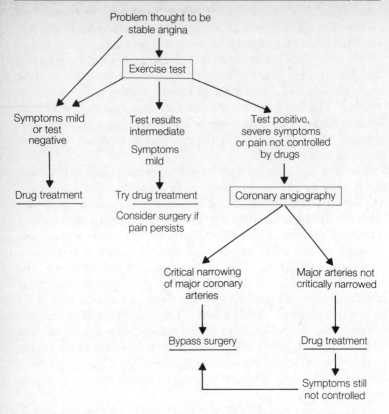

Figure 6.1 'Decision tree' showing possible stages in the diagnosis and recommended treatment of angina.

be referred to a specialist hospital cardiology department for investigation. Here, a likely initial test is the exercise ECG.

When this test shows no evidence that areas of heart muscle are being dangerously deprived of blood, effective control of angina pain is the only important consideration. One of the range of available drugs will usually be prescribed. If the pain is not well controlled, or if there are unacceptable side-effects, other drugs will be tried, on their own or in various combinations. Medical treatment is sufficient to deal with angina in the majority of cases. But when it does not control pain effectively, surgery should be considered. A coronary artery bypass operation would also be advised for patients whose symptoms are rapidly becoming worse despite increased therapy with drugs.

If the exercise test proves positive, it is likely that coronary angiography will be recommended. Figure 6.2 shows three different patterns of coronary artery disease, as revealed by coronary angiography. In all three cases the arteries are dangerously narrowed, and the hearts shown are at serious risk of damage from a heart attack. Figure 6.2a shows narrowing (termed *stenosis*) close to the start of the left coronary artery. This is called 'left main disease'. Where the artery is critically narrowed at this point, coronary bypass surgery significantly improves the patient's chances of long-term survival. Coronary bypass surgery also reduces risk of death when there is severe stenosis in the left anterior descending artery (shown in the second figure), and when all three major coronary arteries are affected by disease (third figure).

Where coronary angiography shows less dangerous patterns of disease, drug treatment that effectively controls symptoms may be completely satisfactory.

Drugs for angina

Any drug that slows the heart rate decreases its demand for energy. A slower beat also means that the heart muscle spends longer each cycle in a relaxed state, which is important, since it is only when the heart muscle relaxes that blood flows into it through the coronary arteries. Drugs that slow the heart also decrease the *force* with which its muscle contracts. This too reduces the heart's requirement for energy. Another way of decreasing the heart's workload is to lower blood pressure. This means that blood pumped out of the heart meets less resistance, so easing the heart's task.

The energy the heart requires is reduced in all of these ways by a class of drugs called the *beta-blockers*, which over the past 20 years have proved one of the most used, and most useful, of all medicines. Beta-blockers lessen the likelihood of angina attacks, but their most widespread function is in the control of blood pressure itself. Details of the range of beta-blocking drugs available, with their particular uses and possible side-effects, can be found in chapter 13.

As their name suggests, *vasodilator* drugs increase the diameter of blood vessels. This encourages flow of blood through the coronary arteries, while at the same time reducing the workload of the heart by lowering blood pressure in the circulation. Vasodilators therefore help prevent angina by acting on both sides of the supply and demand equation. The drugs most commonly associated with angina

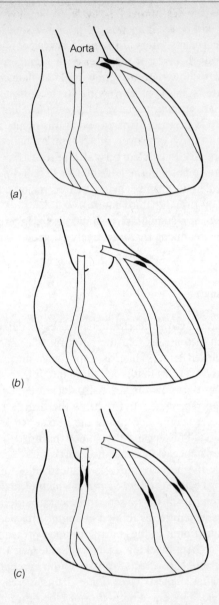

Figure 6.2 Severe narrowing of the coronary arteries at the places shown here means a high risk of serious heart attack, as well as the pain of angina.

are the *nitrate* class of vasodilators, which have provided effective relief from the condition for many years. Whereas drugs like the beta-blockers are taken regularly on a daily basis, and have long-term effects, many nitrate preparations are used for short-term relief of pain or to prevent it when an angina attack is anticipated.

Used in this way, nitrates (such as glyceryl trinitrate, which is also called GTN or TNT) abolish pain within a few minutes, and provide relief from angina for between 20 minutes and an hour. If a nitrate tablet is taken shortly before exercise, the onset of pain can be prevented. Unlike most drugs, these tablets are not swallowed, but dissolved by placing them under the tongue. The drug is then quickly absorbed through the skin lining the mouth. Chewing a tablet brings still more rapid relief. In patients who have infrequent attacks of angina, use of nitrates to control the pain whenever it occurs may be the only therapy needed, though nitrates have the unwelcome effect in some people of producing a thumping headache.

Recently, longer-acting nitrate preparations have been developed, in the form either of tablets that are swallowed or of self-adhesive plasters. (When a plaster is stuck on the chest, the drug is gradually released, allowing its slow but continuous absorption through the skin.) Patients who have angina even when they are not exercising, and those suffering from it at night, may find these slow-release preparations of the drug particularly helpful.

Also relatively new is the use of a group of vasodilator drugs called 'calcium antagonists' or 'calcium-channel blockers'. These drugs act in a number of ways, slowing the rate at which the heart muscle contracts as well as dilating the coronary arteries and blood vessels in the rest of the body. Daily use of calcium antagonists provides long-term relief from angina. Their introduction provides a valuable alternative therapy for those patients who experience unpleasant side-effects (such as nightmares, cold hands and feet, and impotence) with beta-blockers. Calcium antagonists may be particularly helpful in the relatively uncommon situation in which angina is due not to atheroma but to spasm of the coronary arteries.

Further information on medical therapy for angina is found in chapter 13. This section includes chemical and brand names.

Coronary artery surgery

An earlier section has described the thinking that lies behind a doctor's decision to recommend surgery for coronary artery disease.

Broadly, there are two reasons for an operation. One is to relieve pain and improve exercise capacity – and so quality of life – in people whose angina is not adequately controlled by drugs. The other is to reduce the risk of a potentially fatal heart attack when the coronary arteries are likely to become blocked at a crucial point in the heart's blood supply. The usual operation involves bypassing the obstruction in a coronary artery using a small length of vein taken from the leg. The operation is therefore called a coronary artery bypass graft (CABG for short) or a coronary vein graft. In Britain there are more than 6,000 CABG operations each year; in the USA, there are around a quarter of a million.

Such bypass surgery is feasible only because most coronary artery disease occurs in relatively wide parts of the blood vessels near their origin in the aorta. However, atherosclerosis, the 'furring up' of blood vessels that underlies angina and heart attacks, rarely affects one coronary artery alone. One specific obstruction may be responsible for the pain of angina, but the disease almost certainly affects other sites as well.

For this reason, the majority of coronary artery operations involve three or four separate bypass grafts. Where many branches of the coronary artery system are affected, there may be more. Of course not all portions of diseased artery are bypassed. Vessels that are less than 1 millimetre in diameter are usually considered unimportant. There will also be sections of coronary artery that are inaccessible. However, in general, bypasses will be placed around all significant coronary artery branches that have been reduced to half their normal width or less. Where there are too many obstructions to bypass, it may be possible to 'core out' the blood vessel by stripping away its thickened inner lining. This procedure is called *endarterectomy*.

Recently, surgeons have started to favour bypassing diseased coronary vessels using small arteries from inside the chest wall. These procedures are known as internal mammary grafts (or IMAs). In certain cases, they provide a more durable and longer-lasting bypass. However, the most common material used is still vein taken from the patient's own leg. Unless they are varicose veins, these blood vessels usually provide a good substitute for coronary artery. Where the leg vein is damaged or has already been removed, a similar vessel in the arm may be used. The leg has several veins. Removing one of them may cause temporary swelling of the ankle after the operation, but will not have any permanent ill effects.

One end of the vein is sewn over a slit made in the wall of the coronary artery, beyond the point where it is narrowed. The other is attached to a small hole cut in the aorta. The result is shown in figure 6.3. The procedure involves sewing a vein that is no wider than a pencil to a coronary artery that is little larger than a pencil lead, using surgical thread that is about as thick as a coarse hair. To perform such intricate surgery successfully, the surgeon must operate on a heart that is not moving. The heart therefore has to be temporarily stopped. In this period, the heart's function – and that of the lungs – is taken over by a mechanical device known as a heart–lung machine. In technical terms, transferring the job of pumping the blood and supplying it with oxygen from man to machine is known as cardiopulmonary bypass. Making sure that this happens safely is the joint responsibility of the surgeon, the anaesthetist and specially trained technicians who 'man the pump'. (Cardiopulmonary bypass is not to be confused with the *surgical* procedure of bypassing the obstructed blood vessel.) Further details are given in appendix 1 on open-heart surgery.

After the operation

CABG operations generally take between two and three hours. Patients are usually taken to a specialised ward for their early period of recovery, but then transferred after one or two days to a general ward. Most leave hospital in seven to ten days, returning to work in six to eight weeks, with hospital visits once or twice over the next three months for check-up. In some hospitals a check-up will

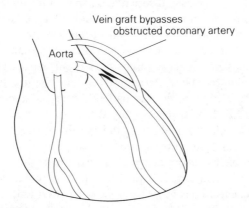

Figure 6.3 In a coronary artery bypass graft (CABG) a piece of vein is used to channel blood directly from the aorta to the coronary artery 'downstream' of the obstruction.

include an exercise test, and may involve coronary angiography to ensure that the bypass vessels have not become blocked and are successfully supplying the heart muscle with additional blood.

Coronary artery bypass grafts reduce angina symptoms and improve exercise capacity in almost all patients. Chest pain is completely relieved in about three-quarters of them. In certain forms of coronary artery disease, the prospects of five and ten-year survival are also significantly improved. Most people who want to return to work do so without problem, though many more elderly patients elect to retire. Those who do go back to their jobs report greater work satisfaction and less fatigue. Family and social life also improve.

Risks and complications

The benefits of the CABG operation are considerable. On the negative side, there is a small risk of death during the operation itself. In most hospitals in the UK, mortality due to the operation is between 1 and 2 per cent. In some it is less. There are many centres in North America, where CABG is even more routine, where the risk of death is around one in 200. As well as the mortality associated with the operation, there is a small risk of a non-fatal heart attack.

There is also the possibility of less obvious forms of damage caused by the operation. Some patients experience minor changes in personality, periods of disorientation and confusion for a few days after the surgery, emotional upsets and difficulties with memory, reasoning and concentration. Many people report visual disturbances, with difficulty in reading, and often complain that TV pictures 'break up'. In most cases, such problems disappear within weeks or months. They are almost certainly due to slight damage caused to the brain while the patient's heart is stopped, and the circulation of blood taken over by the heart–lung machine. Much current research is aimed at minimising this damage.

In the immediate convalescent period, people may experience various problems, many of which are common, but usually short-lived. These include pain and discomfort in the chest associated with the surgical incision. The chest bone (sternum) has of course been cut, and like any broken bone takes eight to twelve weeks to heal completely. During this period occasional physical stresses (such as sneezing) may produce pain; but they will not cause the bone to burst apart. Joints at the ends of the ribs and in the neck and back have also been disturbed during the operation and may be uncomfortable, sometimes for several months. One of the reasons that driving in the first six weeks is advised against is soreness when turning the head. Any infection of the chest wound, particularly of the bone, causes prolonged pain, but this complication is rare. A more common problem, which can be a particular nuisance, is the formation of a raised tender scar, called keloid, where the skin of the chest was cut. Though keloid usually causes discomfort rather than pain, it may be bad enough to delay recovery, and have to be dealt with by specialised plastic surgery.

The leg wound, where the vein was 'harvested', will also be uncomfortable for a while. It may also swell. Patients are therefore recommended to wear support stockings until the leg heals. One of the nerves to the skin of the leg runs close to the vein taken for bypass surgery. Because of this, some patients experience a numbness around the ankle. This lack of sensation may be permanent. As with any major operation, it is quite usual for patients to feel 'out of sorts', and have reduced appetite, a dry mouth and sensations of unpleasant taste, for example. Drugs given after surgery may contribute to these problems, which disappear with recovery and when the drugs are no longer needed.

Certain general problems associated with CABG are similar to those that follow a heart attack. These include coping with being in hospital, controlling anxiety about death and disability, re-adjusting to family life and work, and learning to have confidence once again in the capacity of the heart. These difficulties, and ways of overcoming them, are discussed at length in chapter 5.

Though the development of coronary artery bypass grafting marked a major advance in the treatment of angina, and many patients are elated to be relieved of chest pain, the operation is not a panacea. Angina may recur as disease progresses in blood vessels that have not been grafted; and the bypasses themselves may become narrowed by atheroma. Some form of angina returns within seven years in about 50 per cent of patients. If necessary, the bypass operation can be repeated. The risk of a second operation is marginally greater than that of initial surgery, but is still remarkably safe.

To help reduce the risk of complications after surgery, patients who have had bypass grafts are usually given drugs that reduce the tendency of the blood to form clots. Long-term use of such drugs (which include aspirin and dipyridamole, or Persantin) may also lessen the chances of the bypass becoming clogged once again with atheroma.

The future

Though drugs and conventional surgery are still the mainstay of treatment for angina, our ability to deal with the condition may be revolutionised by new techniques. The use of lasers to burn away atheroma and so clear coronary blood vessels is being attempted in animals. In patients, doctors are already starting to treat angina by pushing a catheter into the coronary artery, then inflating a long thin balloon to squeeze apart the narrowed walls of the blood vessel. This new technique, called coronary angioplasty, and other developments are described in chapter 11.

Reducing the chances of a heart attack

Though many people have a heart attack without previously experiencing angina, there is no doubt that it is a warning sign. According to a study in the USA, which for more than a decade has charted the medical history of thousands of people living in the town of Framingham in Massachusetts, one in four men with angina has a heart attack within five years. (The risk is only half this among women.) Even without changes in lifestyle, and without medical attention, most people with angina live without serious health problems for many years. With appropriate treatment, and prudence, the chances of a full and long life are very good. On average, angina patients now live another ten years, and often survive for twenty.

There is little evidence so far that we can reverse the process by which atheroma forms, though fat that was deposited in the artery wall by blood could conceivably just as easily be picked up by it and removed. After all, the artery is not an inert pipe. Its walls consist of living cells that are constantly interacting with blood constituents.

Removal of atheroma by the body itself, or by drugs, is at the moment no more than a possibility. But every patient has a real chance to reduce the chances that angina will progress to a heart attack. These suggestions apply equally to patients who have surgery and to those whose condition is being treated with anti-angina drugs.

Smokers with angina should stop as the first priority. Compared with non-smokers, smokers are about twice as likely to die from disease of the coronary arteries. One in three 40-year-old men who smoke 20 cigarettes or more a day dies of a heart attack before retirement age. In a patient with lung cancer, there may be very little point in giving up cigarettes. In the case of heart disease, the position is entirely different. It is never too late to benefit from stopping.

Patients with high blood pressure (hypertension) should also take seriously any treatment suggested to reduce it. In people who are overweight, this will probably include some form of diet, as well as drugs. In addition to reducing the quantity of food, it may be wise selectively to reduce the amount of salt and animal fats eaten. Controlling blood pressure is likely to lower the amount of oxygen required by the heart. There is also good evidence that drug therapy for hypertension reduces the risk of stroke. Patients who have diabetes as well as angina may be able to reduce damage to their blood vessels by controlling their sugar levels through careful diet and use of drugs.

It would also be sensible to avoid unnecessary demands on the limited oxygen supply to the heart. Sudden, strenuous exercise, such as pushing a car or shovelling snow, often precipitates severe attacks of angina and may lead to a heart attack. Moderate exercise, however, increases the sense of general fitness and self-confidence. With appropriate use of drugs, it should not bring on angina. There is some evidence that reducing stress by adopting a more leisurely style of life helps prevent the expression of coronary artery disease, and that helpful relaxation techniques can be learned.

Chapter Seven

Abnormal Rhythms of the Heart and Pacemakers

Abnormal heart rhythms – called *arrhythmias* – are relatively common. They arise from disturbances in the electrical conduction system which controls the frequency of the heart beat and the sequence in which its chambers contract. Strictly speaking, 'arrhythmia' means absence of rhythm. For this reason, some doctors prefer to talk of 'dysrhythmias' though most use the words interchangeably.

Many arrhythmias occur in people who have hearts that are otherwise normal, and represent no danger; but others are important symptoms of disease, and some are life-threatening. Abnormal heart rhythms can occur on their own or in association with other heart conditions such as valve, heart muscle and coronary artery disease. Deciding whether a particular arrhythmia is serious or not is often a difficult task. It is made more tricky by the fact that abnormal rhythms may come and go quite suddenly, and are therefore difficult for the doctor to investigate.

Looked at simply, there are potentially two kinds of problem: rate and regularity. The heart can fail to maintain an adequate circulation either because it beats at the wrong speed (which may be too fast or too slow), or because its chambers beat in an unco-ordinated, irregular way. In practice, the two abnormalities are often found together.

The normal adult heart rate varies between around 50 and 100 beats per minute, but may be slower than this in trained athletes, and far faster with exercise, excitement, anxiety and pain. If the heart rate is fast in other circumstances, we speak of palpitations:

the fluttering or thumping sensation in the chest as the heart beats abnormally quickly. People are usually aware of fast arrhythmias – called *tachycardias* – though this is not always the case, even when the burst of fast activity is prolonged.

Normally, as was described in chapter 1, each heart beat starts in a collection of cells in the right atrium called the sinus node. The impulse spreads through both atria, pauses at the AV node, and then passes on to the ventricles (*see* figure 1.6 on p. 12). Thus the collecting chambers beat before the pumping chambers, ensuring that the latter contract only when they have been topped up with blood. However, this orderly, efficient pattern (called sinus rhythm) is often upset. The electrocardiogram (ECG or EKG) is clearly the key to identifying abnormalities of heart rhythm. The ECG trace shows the frequency with which beats are initiated by the heart's pacemaker in the atrium, and charts the passage of the impulse through the rest of the heart.

'Normal' abnormalities

Especially in young people, there is some natural variation in heart rate from beat to beat, since the activity of the sinus node (the heart's natural pacemaker) is affected by the breathing cycle. The heart rate speeds up slightly as we breathe in, and slows as we breathe out. However, this variability is small.

Innocent palpitations

Many people, especially at times of high excitement or emotional stress, feel palpitations. Sometimes these episodes of fast heart rate are made worse by smoking and by tea and coffee, since nicotine and caffeine are cardiac stimulants. Those realising they have attacks may be able to identify specific factors (exercise or drugs like nicotine and coffee, for example) that bring them on. If so, the cause can be avoided. People may also work out ways of stopping palpitations, perhaps by lying down, drinking cold water or holding their breath.

Palpitations generally have a regular rhythm. Usually they cause no significant symptoms, but they may make a person feel weak and faint (and perhaps frightened). Such palpitations may last for seconds, minutes or hours, but rarely for longer. They do not progress to serious forms of disease, and the heart is generally otherwise normal. However, worry about the palpitation may itself make the symptom worse. Where anxiety plays a part, a mild sedative may help.

In medical terms, these episodes are called paroxysmal supraventricular tachycardias (or SVTs): paroxysmal because they are occur suddenly; supraventricular because the fast heart rate originates above the ventricles; and tachycardia, meaning fast heart rate. As we have said, paroxysmal SVTs generally do not need to be treated, though they can usually be controlled by drugs if they prove frequent and disturbing. However, in someone whose heart is *abnormal*, palpitations may tip the balance towards heart failure. In these cases, treatment is required.

'Missed' beats

Sometimes there is a heart rate irregularity that takes the form of an occasional, extra, premature beat inserted between two normal contractions. Such beats are called extrasystoles or ectopics. ('Ectopic', as in a pregnancy occurring not in the womb but in the tubes leading from the ovary, simply means 'in the wrong place'.) Ectopic beats are usually small; and may be too small to be felt. After an ectopic there may be an abnormally long delay before the next contraction, which is often a bigger beat, giving the impresssion that a beat had been missed out. The heart is therefore felt to 'restart' with a thump in the chest.

Ectopic beats are quite common (though often we are unaware of them) and are usually harmless. But there may be problems when they occur frequently, or in 'runs' of several together, or when they originate from abnormal sites in several areas of the heart. These features are signs of more serious underlying disease and require careful diagnosis and treatment.

Investigating abnormal rhythms

The ECG is clearly the most important means of investigating arrhythmias, and the different disorders are defined in terms of their ECG pattern. Taking an ECG is often worthwhile, even when there is not likely to be any serious underlying abnormality of the heart.

Irregular rhythms that persist can quite easily be identified on an ECG trace. However, those that are intermittent are more difficult. One way round the problem is to precipitate an arrhythmia. This can be done quite simply in some circumstances, perhaps by having the patient exercise. In other cases it may require administration of a specific drug, or perhaps the passing of a wire into the heart so that the abnormality can be electrically triggered. Another way of investigating elusive arrhythmias is to equip the patient with a portable ECG machine which records the heart's electrical activity on tape or relays the information to the hospital via a small transmitter. Further information on these and other techniques used in ECG diagnosis can be found in chapter 3.

It is helpful to remember that the same electrical abnormalities can occur in two quite different types of heart: those that are basically healthy, and those that have already suffered from problems such as valve disease and muscle death following a heart attack. Depending on the underlying state of the heart, doctors may suggest quite different ways of tackling what appear to be similar problems.

For problems that arise purely and simply because of abnormalities in the electrical system of the heart, there are two major approaches: the use of pacemakers for heart rates that are too slow, and drug therapy for fast and irregular rhythms. However, if the underlying difficulty is mechanical (for example with the heart valves), a corrective operation may be appropriate. Where the heart muscle is being weakened by inadequate blood supply, bypass surgery may be the answer.

Abnormally fast heart rates

A fast heart rate that maintains a coordinated rhythm is called *sinus tachycardia*. Up to a point, a quick cycle of contraction and relaxation means simply that more blood is pumped. But when working at more than around 160 beats per minute, the heart is no longer pumping efficiently, even if it stays in a regular rhythm, and so the demands of the circulation are not met.

As we have seen, sudden, brief bursts of regular fast activity (palpitations) arising in or around the atria may not need treating. But where tachycardia is persistent, and when fast rhythms are found in one part of the heart but not in others – producing

uncoordinated contraction and so reducing the effectiveness of the
heart pump – treatment is often required.

Since the nervous system is involved in controlling heart rate and
rhythm, it is sometimes possible to regain control of the heart by
simple procedures that stimulate certain nerves. In the case of fast
heart rates that arise in the atria, pressing on a sensitive area in
the neck is sometimes sufficient to restore a normal rhythm. The
technique is called carotid sinus massage.

Fast arrhythmias can make a person feel tired, breathless and
light-headed, as the brain is deprived of oxygen. If blood supply to
the heart itself is reduced, angina may be the result. The same
problem arises if the frantic activity of the heart muscle greatly
increases its *demand* for blood.

Abnormal patterns of heart activity have specific names according
to their site, speed and irregularity.

Fibrillation of the atria

One of the commonest abnormal rhythms (especially in the elderly)
is *atrial fibrillation*. In this condition, the collecting chambers of the
heart beat in an uncoordinated way. Electrical signals from the atria
are transmitted erratically through the AV relay station to the
ventricles, which beat irregularly and also at a higher than normal
rate. This reduces the efficiency of their pumping action, though
the ventricles often manage to sustain an adequate circulation.

People with atrial fibrillation often have abnormal hearts (but the
condition becomes more common with increasing age even when
there is no heart disease). Frequently, the underlying problem is
disease of the mitral valve; but it may be damage to the heart muscle
following a heart attack, or high blood pressure.

Control of the rapid heart rate is usually achieved by taking the
drug digoxin, which slows transmission of electrical signals through
the AV relay station, and so helps protect the ventricles from being
bombarded by unnecessary impulses. Any heart failure that results
from inefficient pumping can be treated with diuretics. (More information about these drugs and their possible side-effects is found in
chapter 13.) With proper medical treatment, most people with atrial
fibrillation can lead normal lives, although some may notice they
are restricted in the amount of exercise they can take.

As blood does not flow freely through fibrillating atria, there is
a tendency for blood clots to form. These can break off and travel

through the circulation, eventually becoming lodged in blood vessels, a process known as *embolism*. Embolism can produce serious complications, such as stroke, if the clots lodge in critical areas. For this reason, many people with atrial fibrillation are given 'blood-thinning' drugs called anti-coagulants. The most common of these drugs is warfarin.

In the condition called *atrial flutter*, the contraction of the collecting chambers is more coordinated than in fibrillation, but it occurs far too fast, at rates of about 300 per minute. Though the ventricles tend to beat at only about half this rate, persistent atrial flutter needs treating. Flutter may develop into fibrillation, and is usually a sign of other forms of heart disease.

Abnormally fast beating of the pumping chambers: ventricular tachycardias

Fast arrhythmias affecting the pumping chambers, called *ventricular tachycardias*, are potentially more serious than those that affect the atria. This is because the main pumping action of the heart is more immediately threatened.

These abnormally fast rates of contraction in the heart's pumping chambers (up to 220 beats per minute) generally reflect existing heart disease, and often follow a heart attack. Ventricular tachycardias cause breathlessness and chest pain, and if untreated may lead to heart failure. They can be reversed by injection of drugs, and future attacks prevented by maintaining drug treatment in tablet form. Electric shocks will also bring ventricular tachycardias to an end. Both forms of therapy are described later.

Ventricular fibrillation

Ventricular fibrillation, which sometimes occurs after a heart attack, is the most serious disorder of heart rhythm. In this condition, the chaotically fast, uncoordinated movement of the heart muscle is best described as 'writhing'. No blood is pumped, the person becomes unconscious and breathing stops. Death follows within minutes if the arrhythmia cannot be reversed by drugs or electric shock, or if the work of the heart is not taken over by some other form of mechanical pumping action, such as the pressure applied to the chest during cardiopulmonary resuscitation (*see* appendix 6).

The treatment of ventricular fibrillation is described below and in chapter 4. The risk of further attacks of ventricular fibrillation can be reduced by long-term treatment with drugs.

General causes of abnormally fast heart rates

Though the heart beat is normally initiated by the sinus node, other groups of heart cells also have the ability to generate electrical impulses. Any abnormal group of cells that produces electrical impulses more frequently than the sinus node stands a chance of 'capturing' heart muscle, making it beat at its own faster rate. Abnormal sources of electrical activity (often referred to as irritable foci) can be found in the atria or in the ventricles.

Another cause is an abnormal circular arrangement of conducting tissue which allows an electrical impulse to 'chase its tail' around an area of the heart, instead of travelling straight through. This phenomenon is known as 'circus movement' (figure 7.1). Such circuits may occur in the atria, the ventricles or in the area of the AV node where collecting and pumping chambers join. The result is an abnormally fast frequency of contraction in the chambers affected.

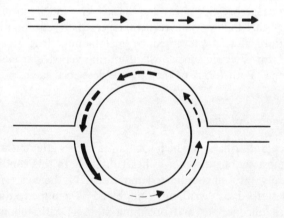

Figure 7.1 In the normal situation (above), regular electrical impulses pass straight through the heart chambers. But where conducting tissue branches and rejoins, there is the possibility the impulse will 'chase its tail'. This is one cause of fast arrhythmias.

This problem can be particularly dangerous in people whose hearts have an extra conducting pathway that joins atria and ventricles but bypasses the AV node. Generally, the AV node acts as a protection for the ventricles, preventing them from being bombarded by abnormally frequent electrical signals generated in the atria. However, abnormal bridges of conducting tissue allow impulses to pass from collecting to beating chambers without the usual delay. Any fast atrial arrhythmia can therefore easily be transmitted straight to the ventricles, causing havoc to the heart's ability to circulate blood. The problem is known as the Wolff–Parkinson–White syndrome (or simply WPW).

Having mentioned these causes of tachycardia, it is worth repeating that many people who experience palpitations have perfectly healthy hearts. Someone who fears they have heart disease may feel their heart beating abnormally fast. The resulting anxiety then itself increases heart rate and can make a problem appear serious when there is little if anything to worry about.

General treatment of abnormally fast heart rates

Fast arrhythmias that start in the ventricles are usually more serious than those in the atria, since the pumping chambers of the heart play the more vital role. Occasional extra beats cause little problem, but continuous fast contraction should be treated.

Many drugs control arrhythmias, but their effective use depends on exact identification of the abnormality involved. Certain drugs are most useful for fast heart rhythms that arise in the atria or around the AV node, while others exert a greater effect on ventricular arrhythmias. The variety of different agents available also offers the opportunity of tailoring therapy to the individual patient. If one drug does not work then another might; if one agent has unpleasant side-effects, another may be free of them, yet just as effective. Finding the drug that best fits a particular person may therefore require patience.

Certain drugs that were initially employed for other forms of heart disease have found an important place in the treatment of arrhythmias. The beta-blockers, for example, can be a part (or the whole) of medical therapy for troublesome tachycardias and ectopic beats, as well as being used in the control of blood pressure and angina. The beta-blockers' effect in slowing the heart may also be valuable in someone whose fast heart rate is the result of anxiety.

xglove drug' digoxin is thought to be the best way of
the ventricles from the effects of atrial fibrillation, as
...ving a stimulant effect on the failing heart (though in too
large a dose digitalis drugs can themselves cause abnormalities of
heart rhythm). Further information about these two classes of drug
is found in chapter 13.

There are other important drugs whose major function is the
control of arrhythmias, and these are mentioned here. They include
the calcium channel-blocker verapamil (Cordilox) which is effective
against fast arrhythmias, and can be injected to stop an attack or
taken in tablet form to prevent them. Among drugs that can be used
in a similar way are disopyramide (Dirythmin and Rhythmodan),
flecainide (Tambocor), mexiletine (Mexitil), procainamide (Pro-
nestyl) and tocainide (Tonocard). All can be used in tablet form as
well as by injection. Lignocaine (Xylocard) is given by injection
only; and quinidine (Kiditard, Kinidin, Quinicardine) is used only
as tablets.

Amiodarone (Cordarone X) is a powerful and relatively new agent
which is used to treat many different arrhythmias. Patients taking
amiodarone may have unusual skin reactions to sunlight. Use of the
drug often produces deposits in the cornea of the eye. These deposits
do not generally affect sight, and disappear once the drug is stopped.
There is a chance that amiodarone will affect the working of the
thyroid gland, and patients taking it for long periods may have their
thyroid hormone levels checked by blood test. Because of these
possible side-effects, amiodarone is rarely the first drug to be tried.
Its long-term use is generally avoided where possible.

When the need is to terminate an arrhythmia, administration of
a brief electric shock offers an alternative to drug treatment. Using
this technique, called *cardioversion*, the heart can be jolted out
of its abnormal rhythm. The treatment can be used to reverse
arrhythmias, such as atrial fibrillation, that may have been present
for weeks or months. It is also valuable in correcting irregularities
that develop in the period following a heart attack. Cardioversion
is described further below.

Some arrhythmias are relatively permanent features of the heart,
and would continue if not treated. In certain of these cases regular
drug therapy may be the only way to prevent the development of
fatal heart failure. Other tachycardias occur infrequently, starting
and stopping unpredictably and of their own accord. People with
these occasional arrhythmias are often free of symptoms such as

giddiness and blackout. They may therefore feel the problem is not worth treating, since having to take drugs daily to prevent occasional attacks is undoubtedly a nuisance. For others, arrhythmias, though they occur only occasionally, affect the circulation enough to cause unconsciousness, and may be life-threatening. For such people, preventive drug therapy may be the sole safe course.

The presence of an abnormal conducting pathway bypassing the AV node is one of the few causes of arrhythmia that can be tackled surgically. It represents an electrical short-circuit in the heart and as such can be broken: a delicate operation to cut the offending tract of tissue resolves the problem. Surgical treatment for this condition (the Wolff–Parkinson–White syndrome is explained on p. 99) is now becoming established. A more recent development involves destruction of the abnormal pathway by delivering an electric shock deep within the heart. This technique is called catheter ablation. Though it has had documented successes, catheter ablation is still at the research stage.

We mentioned above that intermittent but serious arrhythmias may require long-term drug treatment, even though the attacks of tachycardia are few and far between. This situation is far from ideal since anti-arrhythmic drugs are a nuisance to take and may have side-effects (including the small risk that certain arrhythmias will be made worse). Drugs used to treat arrhythmias are often also unsuitable for use during pregnancy. There is therefore great promise in the development of 'smart pacemakers'. These are electrical devices that can be permanently implanted in a patient to monitor the heart rate and correct any abnormally fast activity that occurs. At the moment, though, pacemakers are used almost exclusively for slow heart rates. They are described in the last section of this chapter.

Treating tachycardias after a heart attack

Half the patients in a coronary care unit experience an arrhythmia that affects the ventricles, as 'irritable' areas of tissue around dying heart muscle start to generate their own electrical impulses. Such arrhythmias may not recur once the muscle has healed and formed a scar. But they present a potentially dangerous complication in the first few hours and days of recovery.

Many of these ventricular tachycardias can be treated by intravenous injection of drugs such as those listed above (especially lignocaine), or by delivering an electric shock to the heart through the chest wall. If the ventricles are beating irregularly, but have not yet stopped pumping entirely, administration of an electric shock may wipe out the abnormal patterns of electrical activity that have become established and allow the inbuilt heart rhythm the opportunity to regain control. This technique is called *cardioversion*. The electricity is delivered through 'paddles' applied to the back and chest. Though the shock used is relatively small, it would be uncomfortable, and patients are therefore given a general anaesthetic lasting a few minutes.

The most common cause of death from heart attack is an irregular rhythm of the beating chambers called *ventricular fibrillation*. This represents the most extreme form of tachycardia. Hearts in this condition may as well have stopped altogether for all the blood that is pumped. *Defibrillation* involves jolting the heart into normal rhythm using a large electric shock. A defibrillator is the same device used for cardioversion. Patients needing defibrillation are already unconscious because the brain is not being supplied with blood.

Ventricular fibrillation is an emergency and can quickly be dealt with given the appropriate equipment. But the tendency for a heart to develop ventricular fibrillation may be continuing problem, and require long-term treatment with one of the anti-arrhythmic drugs listed in the previous section.

Slow heart rates

We have mentioned that heart cells possess a natural tendency to beat, and that these rhythms become synchronised when heart cells are grouped together. Cells other than those of the sinus node therefore have the ability to set the pace of the heart. As we have seen, such groups of cells may set an abnormally fast rate, causing tachycardias. But the usual tendency of non-specialist heart cells is to beat at a rate *slower* than those forming the sinus node. The result is that their tendency to beat is normally suppressed.

However, if disease or ageing damages the sinus node so that it fails to generate an impulse, or if the impulse it generates is somehow blocked, other centres set the pace. The first to come into play is a group of cells near the AV node, with an inbuilt rate of around 50 beats per minute. Then come centres in the ventricles themselves, with a natural frequency that is slower still. These subsidiary pace-makers ensure the heart does not stop; but the rhythm they set up is often too slow fully to meet the needs of the circulation. The result is tiredness, accumulation of fluid around the ankles and giddiness. There may also be temporary periods of unconsciousness, caused by insufficient blood reaching the brain, and known as Stokes–Adams attacks.

Analysis of the ECG pattern reveals the cause of the slow heart rate; and doctors talk of different degrees of 'heart block' depending on the site and severity of the problem. A typical case is one in which the atria beat at their normal rate, but the ventricles far more slowly. This situation arises because the sinus node impulse is blocked where atria and ventricles join. Where the cause is inability of the sinus node to initiate a beat, we speak of the 'sick sinus' syndrome. In this condition, both atria and ventricles beat unusually slowly, though there may be periods of abnormally rapid beating as well.

Abnormally slow heart rates are known as *bradycardias*, the Greek prefix 'brady-' meaning 'slow'. Bradycardias sometimes occur because of a birth defect. There is also often a degree of temporary heartblock following a heart attack. This can be treated by a drug, usually atropine, that accelerates heart rate. But the most common cause of bradycardia is a gradual deterioration of the conduction pathways due to ageing. Where treatment is needed, it usually takes the form of an artificial pacemaker.

Pacemakers

When a defect in conduction means that the heart beats too slowly to meet the body's needs, the heart rate can be speeded up using an artificial pacemaker. Used appropriately, pacemakers can transform patients' lives. Through an electrode (usually placed inside the right ventricle itself), a pacemaker directly stimulates muscle contraction at the required rate. In the UK, more than 7,000 pacemakers are implanted each year; in the USA, well over 100,000. Many different types are available, but the principle behind their operation is the same.

There are two parts to a pacemaker: the 'box' that generates the electric pulse, and the wire that conducts it to the heart. In chapter 3, we saw how narrow tubes – called catheters – can be inserted into a vein and pushed gently along until they reach the heart. Insertion of a pacing wire is similar. The wire itself is solid, containing one or two insulated strands. At the tip of the wire, the metal is bare, allowing it to deliver the series of small electric shocks to the heart muscle. The sealed metal pacing box contains a battery as power supply, and electronic circuitry to generate each pulse. This generator weighs a few grams and is a little larger than a box of matches.

Different types of pacing

In the period immediately after a heart attack, a *temporary* pacemaker may be needed to support the rate of the heart. In this case, the pacing wire is usually inserted into a vein at the top of the chest, just below the neck; and the pacing box remains outside the body. Where pacing is to be *permanent*, the wire is fed through to the heart chamber from a generator implanted under the skin between the neck and shoulder (figure 7.2). This involves a small incision (of about 2 in/5 cm). Only a local anaesthetic is required. Though the outline of small, modern pacing boxes can still generally be seen, the generators are usually positioned discreetly enough for their presence to pass unnoticed. With permanent pacemakers, growth of fibrous tissue around the electrode tip firmly keeps it in place within the heart chamber.

In young children, and when the patient is having other forms of heart surgery, the pacemaker electrode may be attached to the *outer* surface of the heart, using a tiny screw. When this is done, the generator box can be positioned in a pouch made between the fat and muscle of the abdomen. Both possible sites are shown in figure 7.2.

Originally, pacemakers simply provided regular electrical impulses, making the heart beat at a constant rate, whatever the heart was inclined to do for itself, but such *fixed-rate* pacemakers are no longer in use. It is preferable to have a more intelligent pacemaker that can sense what the heart is doing and respond accordingly. Such *demand* pacemakers do not fire when the heart generates its own beats, but step in to stimulate a contraction only when they are missed.

Modern pacemakers can generally work in either way, as fixed-rate or demand devices. Use of an electrical gadget called an external programmer enables their mode of working to be switched while

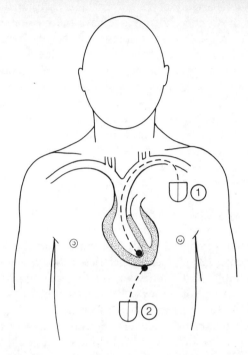

Figure 7.2 Possible sites for a pacemaker. (1) The generaor is placed in a skin pouch near the shoulder, with the electrode lead travelling through a vein into the right ventricle. (2) The generator is in the wall of the abdomen, and the electrode tip attached to the outer surface of the heart.

they are still implanted in the body. The programmer also allows the doctor to alter the rate at which a pacemaker operates, setting it to fire more or less frequently according to the patient's condition. The pacemaker's ability to activate the heart is affected by certain drugs; and the duration and power of the electrical stimulus may need to be adjusted to take this into account.

More sophisticated pacemakers attempt to control not just the rate of beating, but also the *sequence* in which the heart chambers contract. In this way, they aim to simulate the natural production and spread of the electrical impulse through the heart muscle. This usually means that more than one electrode must be placed in the heart: one in the ventricles and another in the atria. These devices produce dual-chambered or 'physiological' pacing. When they are able to sense the activity of the two chambers separately, as well as stimulating them independently, we have the possibility of letting the atria set the pace, while making sure that the ventricles keep in step. This will only work when the sinus node is healthy. But if it is, such pacing means the heart may still be responsive to the body's demands for a faster rate of beating during exercise, for example.

Still 'smarter' pacemakers are able to pick up, process and store information about heart rhythm and make decisions about whether or not to interrupt abnormally fast sequences of beats. The development of these anti-tachycardia pacemakers has been made possible by microchip technology. We return to their potential in chapter 11.

The variety of pacemakers available can produce a confusing picture. A system of classification using a series of letters has therefore been introduced. A VVI pacemaker device, for instance, paces the ventricles (V), senses electrical activity in the ventricles (V), and is inhibited (I) (does not produce an impulse) when the heart produces one of its own. Patients should carry an identity card giving precise details of their pacemaker.

Pacemaker treatment effectively prevents symptoms such as giddiness and fainting attacks, and is helpful however old the patient. In Sweden, 25 per cent of all pacemakers are implanted in people over the age of 80. For someone who has been housebound by such attacks, and the anxiety they provoke, the implanting of a pacemaker can greatly improve quality of life. Generally, the type of device used will reflect the demands likely to be put upon the heart, as well as the underlying problem. So someone who is perhaps younger and more active may require a versatile device, while a simpler form of pacemaker fully meets the needs of an elderly patient. Even when the form of pacing adopted does not allow heart rate to increase with exercise, for example, the heart is able to adapt to the body's greater need for blood by increasing the amount pumped with each beat (*see* chapter 1, p. 9).

Reliability

The lithium batteries powering a modern pacemaker generator should last at least five years, but will eventually need to be replaced, requiring another short operation. Regular check-ups (once or twice a year) at a hospital out-patient department ensure that batteries still have sufficient power and that the device is working well. Nowadays, pacemaker wires break only very rarely.

Demand pacemakers, which can alter their rate, may be sensitive to external electrical signals. Their operation can be upset, for example, by the barriers that screen people at airports and as they leave public libraries. Very occasionally electrical equipment in the home (such as microwave ovens) may also be a problem. Generally, though, the electronics in a pacemaker are well shielded from accidental interference. Doctors who insert the device will have details from the pacemaker's manufacturer about any potential difficulties. Fixed-rate pacemakers are not affected by these potential problems.

Patients who have had a pacemaker implanted successfully and whose symptoms are now effectively controlled should be able to resume driving after a month (*see* also appendix 3).

Chapter Eight

Problems with the Heart's Valves

The need for effective values

On both sides of the heart, there is a valve between the collecting chamber (or atrium) and the pumping chamber (or ventricle). These two valves allow flow of blood into the main pumping chambers. There are also outlet valves between the two ventricles and the major blood vessels – the aorta and the pulmonary artery – into which they pump. Together, the four valves (figure 8.1) ensure the heart pumps blood in the right direction. As the ventricles relax, the inlet valves open and the outlet valves close; as the ventricles contract, the outlet valves open and the inlet valves close. Without them, the heart would not be able to propel blood to the lungs and around the body. (More information about the structure and function of the heart in health and disease is given in chapters 1 and 2.)

The two valves that are most likely to suffer damage are on the left side of the heart, where the ventricle has to pump with greater force . Here, the mitral valve, shown as (1) in figure 8.1, ensures that blood does not flow back into the collecting chamber when the ventricle contracts, and so forces it to leave via the aorta. And the aortic valve (2) ensures that blood pumped out of the heart flows to the rest of the body – and not back into the ventricle when it relaxes to receive the next inflow of blood from the atrium. The equivalent valves on the right side of the heart are the tricuspid valve separating atrium from ventricle (3) and the pulmonary valve (4) separating the pulmonary artery from the ventricle.

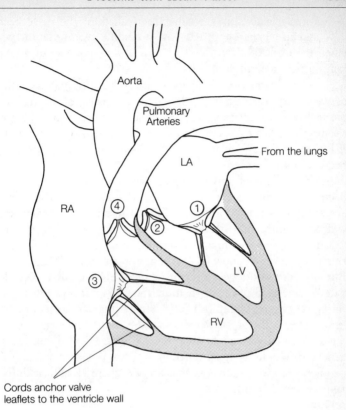

Figure 8.1 The heart valves: (1) mitral; (2) aortic; (3) tricuspid; (4) pulmonary. RA, right atrium; RV, right ventricle; LA, left atrium; LV, left ventricle.

Valve disease and its causes

All valves can suffer from two sorts of problem: the opening through which the blood has to pass can become too narrow; or the valve can leak. The problem of narrowed valves is called *stenosis*; and leakage is termed *regurgitation* or *incompetence*. Though the basic distinction between narrowing and leakage is clear, the reality of valve disease is complex. Many valves are damaged in a way which produces both stenosis and regurgitation – they are like rusty gates that neither open nor shut properly – and patients often have more than one faulty valve.

Stenosis usually arises because the leaflets of the valve become stiff and are later encrusted with calcium. Regurgitation occurs when the leaflets of the valve are torn or weakened so that they no longer form a tight seal.

Valve problems that occur today are frequently the result simply of wear and tear. Though the valves are made of strong fibrous tissue, they are not indestructible when subjected to the strain of opening and closing seventy times and more a minute for a lifetime. With an ageing population, such degenerative valve disease will become more common.

Another cause of valve disease is infection. There are forms of bacteria that colonise heart valves and damage them. Despite modern antibiotics it is occasionally difficult to eradicate these bacteria, and the failure of drug treatment may require prompt surgical repair. The most common source of valve damage in the past – rheumatic fever – is now far less of a problem in the Western world. But surgeons still have to repair or replace valves that have slowly deteriorated as a result of rheumatic fever that occurred twenty or thirty years ago. The mitral valve is particularly affected, and (to a lesser extent) the aortic valve also. Rheumatic fever and its consequences are described in chapter 2. Chapter 2 also considers the general problem of heart infections. This is useful reading since people whose valves are abnormal are at higher risk of heart infection and in certain circumstances may need to take antibiotics as a precaution.

Weakness of the valve leaflets may be caused by a generalised disease of the body's fibrous tissue (in which case the leg and arm joints are likely to be affected). The mitral and tricuspid valves can also be weakened by stretching if the ventricle in which they are set grows larger to compensate for developing heart failure.

The way the leaflets are anchored to the ventricle wall may cause further problems. The leaflets of both valves are normally prevented from 'ballooning up' into the collecting chambers by cords that attach them to the ventricle (figure 8.1). They look rather like the strings of a parachute. If these cords break, or if the muscle that controls them dies when blood supply is cut off in a heart attack, the valve will not seal shut. Stretching of the valve cords is a specific cause of leakage in the condition known as *mitral valve prolapse*. Valves can also be abnormal at birth, though such congenital defects frequently do not cause symptoms until late in life.

Symptoms of valve disease

Since valves are essential to the efficient working of the heart, their malfunction may cause a range of severe symptoms. But this is not always so. Generally, if a valve defect has been slow in developing, the heart adapts to its poor functioning, and symptoms appear only gradually. But if the valve problem develops suddenly, symptoms are serious and may require immediate action.

Taking a specific example of valve disease shows the variety of problems that may arise. From figure 8.1 we can see that severe narrowing of the mitral valve, shown as (1) in the figure, would restrict the flow of blood into the left ventricle and so lead to increased pressure in the left atrium. This causes blood to back-up into the lungs where fluid seeps out of the blood vessels and results in lung tissue becoming stiff. Breathlessness is therefore a possible symptom of valve disease. The problem may appear only when a person exercises or, in more severe cases, also at rest.

Mitral stenosis may also cause palpitations, an awareness of fast or irregular heart beat. Increased pressure of blood in the left atrium strains and damages the atrial muscle. This disturbs the coordinated spread of electrical activity. The atrium therefore beats haphazardly, a condition called atrial fibrillation. Electrical messages pass from the atrium to the left ventricle in an unpredictable way and its regular beating action is therefore also disturbed. (Chapter 7 describes in greater detail abnormal rhythms of the heart and their treatment.)

Angina is thought of mostly in connection with coronary artery disease, but the heart muscle can become short of oxygen and so produce chest pain even when the coronary arteries are not blocked. If the opening of the aortic valve becomes narrowed, the heart muscle has to work harder to pump blood through it. The muscle grows larger, and so may outstrip the ability of the coronary arteries to supply it with blood. There may also be too little blood flowing into the coronary arteries because damaged valves mean the heart is pumping less efficiently.

For the same reason, valve disease sometimes first becomes apparent when a person feels dizzy or faints (though these symptoms have many different causes), since the heart is not pushing out sufficient blood to keep the brain supplied with oxygen. Less serious deficiency of blood and oxygen supply to the body's organs will lead to feelings of malaise and general fatigue.

Valve disease may also be suspected when a patient has a stroke. Blood that is being dammed back behind a poorly functioning valve can produce clots, called emboli, which travel to the brain and obstruct blood supply in places where they become lodged. Because of this risk, patients with valve disease are sometimes asked to take anti-coagulant drugs (such as warfarin) or anti-platelet drugs like dipyridamole (Persantin). Both kinds of drug reduce the tendency of the blood to clot.

Similar damage can be caused to the brain if pieces of calcium break off diseased heart valves and are swept along in the bloodstream. Both forms of emboli may also damage other organs such as the kidneys and bowel.

Aids to diagnosing valve disease

Blood that has to pass through a narrowed opening becomes turbulent and so produces characteristic sounds known as *murmurs*, which can be heard through a stethoscope. The sound of the 'heartbeat' itself also indicates whether valves are working properly since the characteristic 'lub-dup' noise is in fact that of the major valves closing. In some cases the pulse too reveals features suggesting valve disease.

Chest X-rays are important in identifying abnormally large ventricles, which can be either a cause of heart valve problems or one of their effects. (Enlarged ventricles also produce characteristic signs in the electrocardiogram or ECG.) Valves that are encrusted with calcium are sometimes visible on X-rays.

A more useful way of 'seeing' heart valves as they open and shut is by *echocardiography*, in which a moving picture of the heart is built up from reflected sound waves. 'Echo' also identifies abnormally thickened heart-chamber walls. The technique (further explained in chapter 3) uses a principle similar to that of underwater sonar. A refinement of echocardiography, called Doppler, enables the direction of blood flow within the heart to be measured, and provides particularly helpful information in the case of suspected valve disease. Echo, or ultrasound, is fast and involves absolutely no discomfort.

In certain patients more information may be helpful, perhaps to establish the severity of a valve defect and so decide whether an operation is needed. Obtaining this information requires minor surgery (under local anaesthetic) in which measuring devices are passed into the heart using fine tubes called *catheters*. This allows the recording of blood pressure inside the heart's chambers and so provides evidence about the way the valves are working. With stenosis of the aortic valve, for example, pressure in the left ventricle becomes abnormally high as the heart muscle tries to force blood through the narrowed opening.

Catheters are also used to inject the heart chambers with liquid that shows up on X-ray. Liquid that can be seen passing the 'wrong' way through valves is clear evidence they are leaking. These and other sophisticated diagnostic techniques are described in the sections on catheterisation in chapter 3.

Treatment by drugs and surgery

Though much could be done to control symptoms caused by disease of the heart valves, tackling the real problem, the damaged valves themselves, was not attempted until the middle of this century. Then, surgeons developed a way of using a metal rod (or often just a finger) to enlarge the opening in narrowed mitral valves, with the heart still beating.

This valuable operation, called *closed mitral valvotomy*, is still widely used in the developing world. But elsewhere it has largely been replaced by techniques of open-heart surgery in which surgeons stop the heart and operate on it directly. This allows long enough for the full range of damaged valves to be *replaced* as well as repaired. While this is done, a machine temporarily takes over the normal functions of the heart and lungs. (The way the heart–lung machine works is described in appendix 1 on open-heart surgery.)

Replacement valves, also called prosthetic valves, are now basically of two types. Some are mechanical, consisting of a movable metal ball or tilting carbon fibre discs attached to a ring which is sewn in position in the heart. Others are made of tissue, constructed from animal valves (from the pig heart) or the membrane (pericardium) that surrounds the heart of a calf. Mechanical and tissue valves each have their advantages and disadvantages, though both do an effective job. They are considered further below.

Deciding when surgery is needed

Some patients with valve disease are operated on immediately because their lives are threatened by a sudden deterioration in their condition. But for most, the development of the problem is gradual, and many people adapt to the declining efficiency of their heart by limiting their activity. Where symptoms are not uncomfortable, and life is not overly restricted, there is time to consider what to do. In someone who is content to lead a sedentary existence, the need for surgery may never arise. Others, whose quality of life is severely impaired, will consider an operation necessary far earlier in the development of the disease.

Treatment with drugs can help the heart cope better with defective valves, preventing abnormal rhythms and controlling symptoms that develop with heart failure (*see* the sections on drug treatment in chapters 7 and 9). But only surgery can deal with the underlying problem. Deciding when surgery is needed involves estimating likely risks and benefits, and is one of the most difficult decisions doctors and patients have to make. An operation obviously has discomforts and dangers. But doing nothing may also be risky. Faulty valves can deteriorate suddenly; and even slow development of the disease may gradually but irreparably damage the heart to the point where it fails, or becomes too weak to withstand an operation.

If there is a period of 'wait and see', specialists will keep a careful eye on how the valve is working by regular check-ups and occasional admission to hospital for the efficiency of the heart to be tested. Doctors will also be interested in whether the heart is becoming enlarged, since the left ventricle in particular starts to work less well when it is overstretched. Assessment of heart size is usually by X-ray, but has also been greatly helped by the introduction of echocardiography.

Where evidence suggests that the heart is becoming damaged, doctors may suggest prompt surgery even when the patient's symptoms are not severe, and perhaps even when the patient is not aware of any symptoms at all. Where there is severe narrowing (stenosis) of the aortic valve, for example, operations are often needed to protect the heart despite the fact that the patient feels fit and well.

In the case of mitral valve stenosis, the point to watch is the build-up of pressure in the lungs as blood is forced back into the pulmonary veins. There will come a time in the slow development of this disease when the pressure is judged to be reaching damaging levels, and surgery will then be recommended.

Repair or replacement?

Though replacement is now the usual operation for valve disease in the Western world, surgery to repair damaged valves is also possible. As mentioned at the start of the chapter, where the problem is caused by narrowing of the opening, an operation to dilate the valve may be sufficient to delay development of the disease. This is especially so when the mitral valve is affected. In the procedure, called *valvotomy*, a metal instrument (like a closed pair of pliers) is inserted into the valve and then expanded, forcing its sides apart. This operation can be performed without opening the heart or as open-heart surgery, in which case the surgeon can see the valve as he widens its opening. Being able to see the valve directly makes possible more complicated repairs.

If the difficulty arises because blood is leaking through a valve, it may be possible to reduce the size of the opening by inserting a rigid ring. Stitching a tuck into valve leaflets to increase the tightness of their seal can also be tried. Valve *conservation*, rather than replacement, may be particularly helpful in young patients and in pregnant women. There are also many children with congenital heart disease whose malformed valves can be repaired, though this is often only a way of buying time until they are older and valve replacement becomes easier.

Mechanical valves: for and against

Mechanical replacement heart valves are strong, reliable and long-lasting. Rigorous testing simulates the kinds of stresses to be found in the heart and ensures that the risk of mechanical failure is extremely slight. Recent estimates suggest that only one mechanical valve in two thousand will fail. One example (the Starr–Edwards valve) is a metal ball that replaces the action of valve leaflets by moving up and down within a metal cage. Others (for example the

Bjork–Shiley and St Jude prostheses) have a disc or discs that tilt to allow blood to flow past in one direction. Figure 8.2 shows two common types of mechanical valve.

A distinct disadvantage of mechanical valves is that blood flowing over the artificial surfaces tends to form tiny clots which may later block blood vessels. To prevent this, patients who have implanted mechanical valves must take drugs that reduce blood clotting (anti-coagulants) for the rest of their lives. The drug most commonly used is warfarin. The extent to which these drugs are working needs to be checked regularly at anti-coagulation clinics.

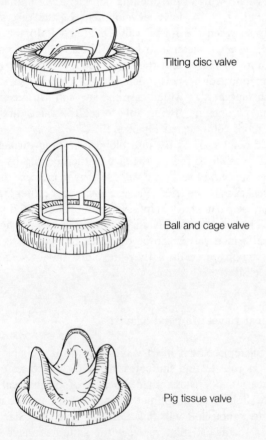

Tilting disc valve

Ball and cage valve

Pig tissue valve

Figure 8.2   Three types of artificial valve.

Apart from the personal inconvenience, and the expense, anti-coagulant drugs mean that blood may not form the clots needed to prevent its loss from wounds. This can be troublesome, especially where people are exposed – perhaps at work – to risk of serious accidental injury.

In pregnancy, women run the additional risk that anti-coagulant drugs may harm their unborn child. These drugs cross the placenta, and significantly increase the chances of abortion – though the likelihood that a child will be born malformed is not great. A final disadvantage is that both the caged ball and tilting-disc varieties of mechanical valve make a ticking noise which people with such implants are often asked to explain.

Tissue valves: for and against

The alternative to metal or carbon is to make a substitute valve from animal material. These are of two types: an actual aortic valve taken from a pig (which will replace either our aortic or our mitral valves); or a tissue valve fashioned from three leaflets cut from the outer sac (pericardium) of a calf's heart. The Hancock, Carpentier–Edwards and Wessex are common makes of pig valve. One is shown in figure 8.2. Any animal tissue is treated to make it biologically inert so that our bodies do not recognise the material as foreign and try to reject it.

Natural, animal-tissue valves overcome the problem of coagulation. There is therefore little risk that harmful blood clots will form, and (except in certain circumstances, such as when there is a risk of atrial fibrillation) there is usually no need for the lifetime use of anti-coagulant drugs. This advantage may be especially important for young women who want to have children.

Animal valves are effective and tend to be more expensive. But they wear more quickly than mechanical implants, may rupture under the continuous strain of working in the left ventricle and tend to become clogged by the accumulation of calcium and a blood constituent called fibrin. In growing young children, tissue valves wear particularly quickly and so are generally not suitable. The same is true for patients who have kidney failure.

Generally, people given tissue valves must expect they will need a second operation. The risk of complications, though not large, rises with each operation. But, overall, it may be no greater than the additional risks of taking anti-coagulant drugs for many years. These points show there is no ideal substitute for human heart valves; and the choice between mechanical and tissue replacements is often not clear-cut. Doctors will advise on the valve they think is best suited to the individual patient.

Living with an artificial valve

Though artificial valves are extremely reliable, there are certain common-sense precautions. Most important, anyone given drugs to reduce blood coagulation must make sure they take them regularly. They must also attend the hospital whenever asked to have their blood clotting time measured. In case they are involved in an accident, patients taking anti-coagulant drugs should carry with them at all times a card giving details of the drugs they are on.

Secondly, anyone with an implanted valve who feels unwell should not hesitate to go to the doctor. Artificial valves slightly increase the risk of heart infections. People who have them should therefore take the precautions mentioned in chapter 2. And there is always the very small chance that the valve will fail. If the implanted valve is mechanical, any change in the noise it makes should quickly be checked.

Chapter Nine

Support for the Failing Heart

For any number of reasons to do with the valves of the heart, its rhythm or the state of its muscle, the heart may begin to fail: that is, it becomes unable to circulate blood effectively enough to meet the demands of the body. Where the underlying cause is a valve defect, it can often be repaired; where the problem is one of arrhythmia, the electrical abnormality can frequently be controlled using drugs or an artificial pacemaker. In people who have abnormally high blood pressure, demands on the heart are increased; and failure occurs earlier than it otherwise would have done. Controlling hypertension can therefore be important treatment for the failing heart. However, there are many cases of heart failure in which it is difficult to remedy the real problem. Most commonly this lies in deterioration of the heart muscle caused by coronary artery disease and so lack of oxygen supply. Infection can also lead to permanent damage to the heart muscle (*see* chapter 2), though this is a far rarer problem.

Mild heart failure following a heart attack is often short term, and responds to medical therapy. Where mild heart failure persists, the heart may itself be able to adapt, so that a person's lifestyle is little affected, though the condition may slowly deteriorate over many years. In a few patients with certain forms of severe heart failure, the development of transplantation (discussed in chapter 10) has brought the chance of cure. However, in the majority of cases, doctors can offer relief of symptoms. The variety of drugs available means that many people have their heart failure kept well under control for years. But in the most severely affected patients, long-term heart failure becomes incapacitating, despite the best available treatment with drugs.

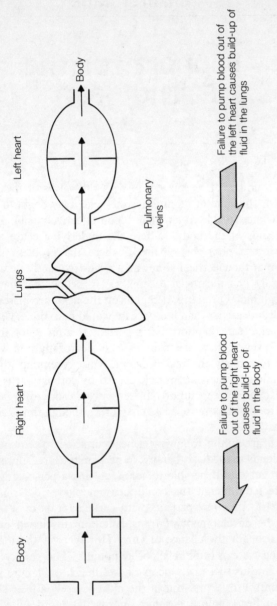

Figure 9.1 The problem of heart failure.

Pumping problems

As we saw in chapter 1, the right and left sides of the heart each act as pumps, the right ventricle pumping blood to the lungs and the left ventricle serving the rest of the body. Frequently, failure affects both sides of the heart. However, the two pumps may be separately affected.

When the *left* side of the heart fails, breathlessness is particularly characteristic. In this condition, the weakened left ventricle cannot pump sufficient blood out of the heart. This leads to accumulation of blood in the left atrium, which in turn restricts flow of blood out of the lungs (figure 9.1.) Pressure in the pulmonary veins therefore increases and the liquid element of blood is forced through the blood vessel walls into the tissues of the lung itself. Lungs clogged with water in this way become stiff, it is difficult for them to expand and deflate and the exchange of oxygen for carbon dioxide is reduced. The chest feels tight, and the person affected is breathless. These problems are made worse even by mild exercise.

Similar principles account for the difficulties that appear with failure of the *right* heart. When the right ventricle cannot pump effectively, blood is dammed back in the right atrium and then in the body's veins as it seeks to return to the heart. Leakage of fluid out of the veins builds up in body tissues giving them a 'puffy' appearance, and causing swelling (oedema) at the ankles. The liver and abdomen also swell, and the gut feels congested, leading to loss of appetite.

To explain what happens in heart failure, we have discussed the two sides of the heart as separate pumps. In fact, heart failure often affects both: poor pumping performance by the left ventricle itself leading to developing failure of the right heart. A generally inadequate circulation also impairs the working of the body's other organs. Among them are the kidneys, which (in addition to other tasks) have the job of excreting sodium (salt) in the urine. When the kidneys are unable to excrete enough, levels of sodium rise. Sodium retained in the body tends to retain water also, contributing to the build-up of fluid in the blood and so its leakage into lung and body tissues. Worsening oedema leads to fatigue, feelings of being generally unwell, breathlessness and a still greater strain on the heart. If the condition cannot be reversed, there is a downward spiral leading to complete collapse of the circulation.

Rest and other treatments

In someone who is very elderly, and unlikely to make major demands on their heart, there may be little need for treatment. In others too, rest can play a part in controlling symptoms, at least in the short term. Exercise causes rapid return of blood to the right heart, which then pumps it into the lungs, from where it flows into the left atrium and ventricle. When the left ventricle is unable to deal with this increased flow, blood backs up into the lungs and breathlessness becomes worse. For someone with left heart failure, sitting may be more comfortable than lying down, even for sleep. This is because gravity causes blood to 'pool' in the veins of the lower body. Less blood returns to the heart, so there is less to accumulate in the lungs, and leakage of liquid into its tissue is reduced.

The problem of heart failure is frequently short term, requiring support for a brief period while the underlying cause is remedied or the heart itself allowed to recover. There are often a few days after heart surgery, for example, when the heart needs help, but is then able to work on its own. A heart attack may lead to similar difficulties for a short period. Treatment in these cases is usually by drugs, though devices that mechanically assist the heart's pumping action may also help. Since such patients are in hospital, the drugs are frequently given by injection or slow infusion into a vein.

Where the underlying problem cannot be resolved, heart failure may mean long-term therapy with drugs. This happens particularly with people who have had a major heart attack, or whose heart muscle has been damaged by a series of smaller infarcts. There are a variety of complementary approaches to drug treatment. Alone or in combination, they are usually sufficient to provide effective relief from symptoms.

Drugs for heart failure

In heart failure, the ventricles have difficulty in circulating blood around the body and lungs. Broadly, there are three classes of drug that may help in this situation. First, there are drugs that make the heart pump with greater force. Secondly, there are those that reduce the workload of the heart by lowering the total *amount* of blood in circulation. Thirdly, there are those that expand the blood vessels. This reduces the *pressure* of blood in the circulation, so that the ventricles have to work less hard to pump blood out of the heart. These three strategies are portrayed in figure 9.2.

Digitalis drugs: making the heart work harder

In 1785, a Birmingham doctor called William Withering described how the heart could be made to pump with greater force using a preparation of foxglove leaves first shown to him by 'an old woman of Shropshire'. In the 200 years since then we have been unable to find a better drug to replace the foxglove. Its extract, digitalis (or the man-made equivalent digoxin, most commonly prescribed as Lanoxin) is still one of the major treatments for heart failure. (Digitalis drugs are also discussed in chapter 13.)

It is generally agreed that digitalis drugs have a mildly stimulant effect on the heart, though its true worth is now much debated by

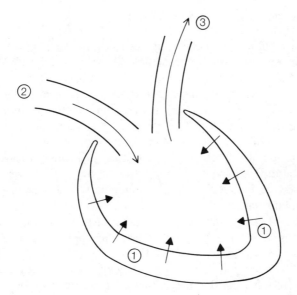

Figure 9.2 Ways of using drugs to help heart failure. (1) Increase the force with which heart muscle pumps; (2) reduce blood *input* to the heart; (3) relieve pressure on the flow of blood out of the heart.

doctors, especially since digitalis is known to have frequent and unwelcome side-effects. One problem is that the dose at which the drug has a beneficial effect is only a little lower than the dose at which its toxic action starts to appear. Another is that (in certain patients at least) its beneficial effects appear to wear off after a few weeks.

Where heart failure is accompanied by a particular disorder of heart rhythm (atrial fibrillation, in which the collecting chambers beat abnormally fast), digitalis is still generally acknowledged to be the most effective treatment. In this condition, digitalis works particularly well because of its influence on electrical conduction in the heart rather than because of its stimulant effect on heart muscle.

In hospital, heart failure can be treated by the injection of a variety of drugs that stimulate the pumping action of the heart more powerfully than digitalis. However, these drugs are not effective in tablet form and so cannot be given outside hospital. Much research effort is being devoted to the development of effective cardiac stimulant drugs (called inotropes) that can be taken by mouth.

Reducing the volume of blood: diuretics

In cardiac failure, the heart is unable to supply sufficient blood to meet the demands of the circulation. If we cannot always restore the balance by making the heart work harder, we can at least attempt to lower the demands placed upon it. Diuretics relieve the workload of the heart by reducing the amount of fluid in circulation. They do this by increasing the excretion of sodium and so the flow of urine – hence their popular description as 'water tablets'. Diuretics are also frequently used to treat high blood pressure.

Several different types of drug have a diuretic effect, varying in their speed and strength of action. Common varieties are frusemide (Lasix), bumetanide (Burinex) and bendrofluazide. Others are listed in table 13.3 (*see* p. 168). Certain diuretics lead to loss of potassium (as well as sodium) in the urine. Potassium supplements may therefore need to be taken (*see* p. 167).

The discovery of diuretics has largely replaced treatment by removal of salt from the diet, which used to be a standard therapy for heart failure. However, patients are still strongly advised to reduce their intake of salt. Avoiding the addition of salt to food at table and keeping clear of salted snacks are good ideas.

Expanding blood vessels: vasodilators

Lowering the overall amount of blood in circulation, which is the effect of the diuretic drugs just discussed, is one way of easing the heart's job. Another is to lower the *resistance* to the pumping action of the heart, and to *redistribute* blood away from it. This is done by drugs called vasodilators.

The body's natural response to heart failure is to constrict the arteries. This is a useful reaction if the underlying problem is loss of blood, but otherwise tends to make the position worse since it is far more difficult for a pump to circulate fluid when the tubes in the system are narrowed and so offer a high resistance to flow. A major aim in treating heart failure is therefore to reverse the body's natural response and *expand* the blood vessels. Hence the usefulness of vasodilators.

Reducing the resistance against which the heart has to pump is one way of easing its task. Another is to lower the amount of blood it has to pump. As we have seen, diuretics have this effect by increasing excretion of fluid. Vasodilators produce the same effect, but via a different mechanism. By expanding the blood vessels – in particular the veins – more blood is kept 'pooled' in the body, and less returns to the heart. Certain vasodilator drugs work predominantly by expanding the arteries, and others by expanding the veins; but most affect both sides of the circulation.

A drug called nitroprusside quickly and effectively dilates blood vessels and so relieves pressure on the heart, but can only be given by injection. However, there are long-lasting tablet preparations of certain nitrate drugs used to treat angina; and these may be helpful in the long-term control of heart failure. They include GTN or TNT (glyceryl trinitrate) and isosorbide dinitrate. More details of these preparations are given in table 13.4 (*see* p. 170).

Other vasodilator drugs that can be taken in tablet form include prazosin (Hypovase) and hydralazine (Apresoline), both of which are also used to reduce blood pressure. In addition, there are two increasingly important new agents – captopril and enalapril – to help with long-term problems caused by a failing heart (*see* the section on ACE inhibitors in chapter 13).

Often, patients with heart failure are given a diuretic (with or without digoxin) as a first attempt to control the condition. If problems continue, it may be necessary to add a vasodilator. With appropriate combinations of drugs and careful choice of dose, most people with mild and moderate heart failure can live a perfectly normal life.

Treating heart failure in hospital

When heart failure needs to be treated in hospital, the pattern of care depends on the severity of the condition. Many patients simply need their drug treatment adjusting, or perhaps require a different combination of drugs. Such 'fine-tuning' of therapy often requires the skills of a specialist cardiologist. Others, who have heart failure that develops suddenly or whose condition is becoming worse, may need more intensive monitoring and treatment. On occasions this is best done in an intensive care unit (or ICU).

The general approach involves bed rest and careful observation. Since oedema is a major problem with heart failure, the intake and output of fluids will be closely controlled. This may mean restrictions on the amount drunk, and measurement of urine passed. A patient's weight will also be watched. Clinical signs such as blood pressure and the state of veins in the neck will be monitored. Regular chest X-rays may be needed to check for fluid in the lungs.

Drugs

We mentioned that digitalis (digoxin) makes the heart work harder, and that similar drugs which increase the force of heart muscle contraction are called inotropes. In the healthy state, this job is done by the body hormones adrenaline and noradrenaline. However, these two substances have many effects, certain of them clearly a disadvantage when the heart is already under stress. So attempts have been made to find drugs that are more precise in their action. Two important drugs that mimic the body's natural mechanism for stimulating the heart are dopamine and dobutamine. They cannot be used in tablet form and are only given intravenously to people with heart failure in hospital. The range of vasodilator and diuretic agents already described is also used.

For safety and convenience, drugs are often administered through a tube (or 'line) permanently positioned in a patient's vein. This allows drugs to be quickly injected – generally producing a fast effect – or more gradually infused. Either way, the dose administered and its effects on the body can be precisely controlled.

Monitoring heart function

Where severe heart failure is being treated in hospital (perhaps as one of the complications following a heart attack), doctors will usually want to know exactly how the heart is performing. The clinical observations described provide certain information; but to judge the best form of therapy – and to assess its effects – it may be necessary to insert measuring instruments into the heart itself. This is done using the fine tubes (or catheters) described in chapter 3.

Among the most useful instruments is a Swan–Ganz or 'balloon catheter'. This device is inserted into a vein in the arm and guided into the right side of the heart. There the balloon is inflated, and the tube carried by the flow of blood into the lungs, where it eventually becomes lodged. The pressure at the balloon tip provides a good indication of how well the heart is working. By injecting a cold solution through the catheter, and monitoring temperature change 'downstream', doctors can also calculate exactly how much blood the heart is pumping. (This is called the cardiac output.)

Mechanical devices to help the heart

Since the failing heart is essentially just a pump that is in trouble, it ought to be possible to develop mechanical devices to assist its working. So far the only device which has proved at all effective is a 'balloon pump', which is positioned in the aorta, the large vessel that takes blood from the left ventricle to the body. The balloon has a dual action: it deflates when the heart contracts, so that the muscle of the left ventricle has to work less hard to pump out its contents; and then the balloon expands as the heart relaxes, increasing pressure in the aorta and so encouraging blood to flow into the openings of the coronary arteries. The device is sometimes used to provide temporary support following open-heart surgery, and is occasionally tried in patients who have severe heart failure following a heart attack. However balloon pumping is not widely used.

Other devices are in the research stage. These include pumps to take over part of the heart's job or all of it, as in the implantable artificial heart described in chapter 11. Such pumps may one day be effective enough to maintain the circulation until arrangements can be made for transplantation. But they are unlikely to provide a long-term solution to problems of heart failure.

Chapter Ten

Heart Transplants

For people who are severely affected by certain forms of heart disease, a transplant can now both extend life and improve its quality. Eighty per cent of patients given 'new' hearts can expect to survive one year; and it looks as if more than half will still be alive after five. Average life expectancy without the operation seems to be around nine months. A heart transplant is thought of as a severe test of a patient's resilience. But there seems little doubt among people who have had the operation that it was worthwhile.

How are patients selected?

Transplanting a heart is a major step for surgeon and patient alike, and selecting those people who will benefit most is carefully done. Patients and their relatives usually come to the hospital for an assessment period. This provides time to discuss potential problems and anxieties, and allows patients to meet those who will care for them.

Transplants are only considered for people whose hearts are diseased beyond possibility of cure using drugs or other forms of surgery. Most patients are already suffering from severe heart failure. Many have heart muscle which has been catastrophically damaged by lack of oxygen supply. Often they have had a series of heart attacks. Others have suffered from rare infections (or from other, often unknown factors) that cause irreversible deterioration of heart muscle.

The results of heart transplantation are best if a patient's general state of health is likely to be reasonably good after the operation.

This means it is generally not suitable for the elderly (in the UK patients older than 60 years do not have transplants), nor for people with other medical problems, such as kidney and liver disease. In the early years, patients had to be psychologically robust to withstand the rigours of recovery; but as transplantation has become more routine, this is now seen as less important.

The operation

As a surgical procedure, heart transplantation is not especially difficult. After the 'old' heart is removed, it takes only four joins to sew the 'new' heart in place. On average this stage takes only 45 minutes. But the whole operation may require three to five hours. Many of the procedures are similar to those involved in any open-heart surgery, and are described in appendix 1.

Hearts can be reliably preserved for up to four hours using protective solutions and by packing them in ice. They can therefore be transported long distances to the hospital where the recipient is waiting. However, it is important to avoid any unnecessary delays: finely coordinated timing is therefore required.

Postoperative care and preventing rejection

People who have had a transplant often recover quickly since they now have a properly functioning heart. Patients generally stay in hospital for three to five weeks. For the first few days they are intensively monitored in highly specialised units, and then transferred to more general wards. To shorten hospital stay, certain transplant centres have hostel accomodation nearby. This also allows patients to make a gradual return to the community. Once home, they are seen monthly by their own doctor, and yearly for a checkup at the hospital where the transplant took place.

The factor that makes transplantation more difficult than other surgery is the possibility of rejection. The body's protection against disease is the immune system which recognises cells that do not belong to us (or are abnormal) and then mobilises defences against them. A heart that has come from someone else is quite properly regarded by the immune system as 'foreign', even though in this instance it poses no threat. The resulting attempt to get rid of the foreign tissue leads to the process of rejection. This damages the heart, causing it to swell and stop pumping efficiently, and has led to many deaths.

In 1980 a new anti-rejection agent, cyclosporin A, was introduced. In combination with other drugs, cyclosporin effectively controls rejection and has been a major factor in greatly improving the success rate of heart transplantation, though balancing drug therapy against risk of rejection in the critical first three months is still a tricky procedure.

For patients simply to survive is not enough. They must have a quality of life that makes survival worthwhile. Recent research from Papworth and Harefield Hospitals, Britain's first two transplant centres (which together have now performed several hundred operations), confirms that this is achieved. Before the operation, patients rated their quality of life at between 0 and 4 on a scale of 0 to 10; after transplantation, these scores were between 8 and 10. People who had been confined to bed and lost almost all their social contacts were able to resume full lives. Transplant patients do not see themselves simply as less ill than before the operation; they score the same on the quality of life scale as people of similar age from the general population. One year after operation, between half and two-thirds of heart transplant patients had returned to work. Before the operation, only one in ten had been able to work.

Future prospects

Since 1980, heart transplants have become far more common; and, especially in the USA, transplant centres are proliferating. For every million people in the population, it is estimated there are ten each year who would benefit from heart transplantation. Half are people whose hearts have been so scarred by lack of blood supply that they no longer pump effectively. Most of the remainder have other disorders of heart muscle.

Despite current success – sufficient for doctors to talk now of heart transplantation having come of age – there are still difficulties. One is the reliable, early detection of signs that the body is rejecting the implant. At the moment, the only way this can be done is by passing a fine tube into the heart itself, to obtain a small sample of tissue for examination under a microscope. In the future it may be possible to detect rejection from blood samples or by imaging the heart using ultrasound.

There are also continuing difficulties in treating rejection. Cyclosporin is a great improvement on previous drugs (notably the steroids), but has adverse effects on the kidney and causes high blood pressure in most patients. Though it prevents rejection in a way which does not completely knock out the body's immune defences, the transplant patient is undoubtedly more susceptible to infection. In some cases the viruses and parasites that cause the problem are probably present in the transplanted organs themselves.

The fact that heart transplant patients are living so much longer has also made us aware of the risks of disease in the 'new' heart. Patients with transplanted hearts tend to develop atheroma deposits along the coronary arteries. The condition (which may itself be a form of rejection) tends to develop quickly and affects many small blood vessels, which means that coronary bypass grafts are not a suitable treatment. When severe enough, this 'furring up' of the blood vessels can cause heart attack. (Interestingly, it does not cause angina, since transplanted hearts have no nerve connections.) Long-term use of drugs such as low-dose aspirin and dipyridamole (which reduce the tendency of blood platelets to clump together) may counter the problem.

The availability of donor hearts for transplantation used to be the major difficulty. This is no longer the case in the UK. People realise the life-saving nature of a transplant, and increasingly accept that in case of death their own organs and those of their relatives should be used. Early (and misplaced) concern that patients would have organs removed before they were truly dead has now been dispelled.

However, performing a transplant requires enormous organisation. The donor heart has to be matched with a recipient who is likely to provide the most favourable new environment; the heart has then to be transported under difficult conditions to the site of the operation; and the aftercare of transplant patients is still complicated, despite greater experience and new techniques. The result is that scarcity of resources is often the limiting factor. Each transplant costs around £13,000 for the first six months, and £2,000–3,000 each year after that for continuing check-ups and drug therapy. This amount of money may seem large, but compares favourably with other kinds of treatment in terms of the benefits that patients derive. There are hearts that could be used, and patients who need them; but not yet sufficient facilities to allow the operations to go ahead.

Combined heart and lung transplants

In 1981, surgeons in California led by Bruce Reitz began a series
of combined heart–lung transplants. The operation was first performed in Britain three years later. There have now been several
hundred such operations worldwide, and the first results suggest
that between 60 and 70 per cent of patients are alive one year later.

Disorders of the heart frequently lead to excessively high blood
pressure in the lungs, causing irreversible damage. Replacement of
both organs is therefore needed. Heart–lung transplants are also the
only effective treatment for certain birth defects which can be
improved long enough for patients to reach adulthood but which
cannot be cured by other forms of surgery.

Finding a suitable donor for a combined heart and lung transplant
is difficult, since as well as the usual requirements the organs have
to be very similar in size to those they are to replace. Diagnosing
rejection early is also tricky, because the heart and lungs can be
separately affected.

Lungs are easily damaged during removal and transport before
the operation. Once they have been transplanted, they have to be
particularly carefully checked for infection; and they may deteriorate
with time. Although still at its developmental stage, early results
with the combined heart–lung operation are encouraging.

Chapter Eleven

The Future

Heart attacks are clearly the most important problem in heart disease. Roughly 50 per cent of the quarter million that occur in Britain each year are fatal. So, if we are really to make an impact on death and disability, it must be done by improving our treatment of this condition. Whatever the long-term factors that increase risk, it is now generally agreed that the immediate cause of a heart attack is the formation of a clot – called a thrombus – that blocks a coronary artery. One hope is that we will be able to find an easily-administered and safe drug that dissolves the clot and so restores the flow of blood. If this is done, heart muscle can be prevented from dying.

Drugs to dissolve clots

Several substances that dissolve clots (a process called *thrombolysis*) have recently been used in clinical trials in America and Europe. Patients arriving in hospital with a heart attack were assigned at random to receive either the new treatment with thrombus-dissolving drugs or conventional therapy. (Such carefully controlled comparisons are the only way to provide objective evidence that a new treatment is superior to the old.)

The first results are promising. It looks as if there are fewer deaths among patients given the new thrombolytic drugs. It also seems that less cardiac muscle dies. This can be shown by measuring the amount of enzyme released into the blood by dead heart cells. Since more muscle is spared to power the pumping chambers,

damage to the efficiency of the heart should also be less, and there
is some evidence this is the case.

However, there are several limitations to the widespread use of
thrombolytic therapy. To have maximum effect on the clot, it is
best to inject the drug straight into the affected coronary artery

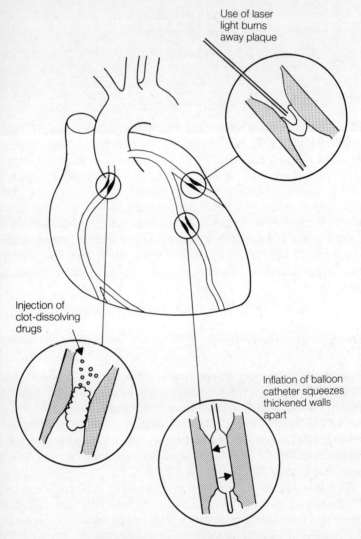

Use of laser
light burns
away plaque

Injection of
clot-dissolving
drugs

Inflation of balloon
catheter squeezes
thickened walls
apart

Figure 11.1 Clot-dissolving drugs, angioplasty and lasers: new and possible
ways to tackle the immediate cause of heart attack.

(figure 11.1). But finding which artery is blocked, and then delivering the drug directly to it, means that the patient must undergo cardiac catheterisation: a fine tube must be inserted into an artery and eased along until it reaches the heart. (The way this procedure can be used to map coronary arteries is described in chapter 3.)

Cardiac catheterisation can only be done in major hospitals; and it carries a small but definite risk. Most important of all, it takes time. The best estimate we have is that heart muscle deprived of blood is irreversibly damaged within four hours. Since most people take an hour or so to realise that they are having a heart attack, and are then inevitably delayed in getting to hospital, there is little time to spare for catheterisation.

There is therefore much to be said for a thrombolytic drug that can be given in the home or on the street. Preferably it should be safe enough to be administered to almost anybody by ambulance or other paramedical personnel. Such a drug would have to be injected into a vein, probably in the arm. It would therefore be diluted throughout the body and have to be given in large doses to have any effect on a faraway clot. As a way of getting the drug to its target thrombus, giving it intravenously has been compared to transporting a chemical from Oxford to London by tipping it into the Thames. The other problem is that the clotting mechanism in the body as a whole would be disrupted, with a risk of bleeding complications, for example in the stomach and intestine.

Attempts are being made to devise forms of thrombolytic drugs that are clot-specific. That is, they are activated *only* when they become attached to fresh thrombus. Two agents promising in this respect are a form of the enzyme streptokinase, and a compound called tissue plasminogen activator (TPA). TPA is naturally present in our bodies in tiny amounts, but can be produced in large enough quantities by genetically engineered bacteria to be used as a drug. It is too early yet to say whether either substance will fulfill its potential as a 'magic bullet' to be used at the first signs of a heart attack.

Even if such drugs hit their target, and leave other parts of the body undamaged, we will still find that chemically dissolving the coronary artery clot is not enough. Blood vessels that have been successfully reopened show a tendency to become blocked again, often within a few weeks, even though patients are given agents that discourage clotting. Drug therapy therefore clearly needs to be backed up by *mechanical* intervention to relieve the narrowing that gave the clot the opportunity to obstruct the artery in the first place. Techniques of widening narrowed blood vessels are called angioplasty. Various methods are being tried.

Balloon angioplasty

One procedure involves inflating a tiny balloon inside the partly obstructed artery, forcing the fatty deposit back into the blood vessel wall (figure 11.1). The technique was first used successfully to treat obstructions in the arteries serving the legs. Balloon angioplasty for coronary arteries was begun in 1979 and is becoming routine in the USA, where there are now 60,000 such procedures each year. Balloon angioplasty also has enthusiasts in Britain, who last year performed 2,500 operations.

Balloon angioplasty begins in the same way as any cardiac catheterisation. The fine tube is manoeuvred along a major blood vessel from the arm or leg until it reaches the opening (at the base of the aorta) of the affected coronary artery. In a further feat of virtuoso navigation, the catheter is eased along the artery until the section containing the balloon lies astride the narrowed section of blood vessel. Liquid is then pumped into the balloon until it is fully expanded, splitting the hardened atheroma deposit and crushing it against the artery wall. Balloon inflation usually lasts 15–30 seconds, using a pressure of four or five atmospheres. The supply of blood through the artery is of course completely blocked for a brief period, but the heart muscle seems to tolerate this temporary situation without complaint.

In a sense, balloon angioplasty is crude, since the technique undoubtedly damages the delicate artery wall. However, drugs are given to reduce the tendency of blood to clot and to limit the clumping of platelets; and removal of the balloon generally leaves the expanded vessel intact.

In the majority of cases, balloon angioplasty has a long-term beneficial effect on blood flow. But in around 30 per cent of patients, narrowing of the affected artery recurs, often at the same point. When this is going to happen, it usually does so within six months. If re-stenosis occurs, balloon angioplasty can be repeated. The procedure is part of the follow-up treatment for patients who have been given thrombolytic drugs. As such, it can be seen as alternative to surgery to bypass the obstructed coronary artery, which patients may be offered after a heart attack.

Balloon angioplasty is also being advocated as a treatment for angina in patients whose symptoms are not controlled by drugs. In people with this problem, the balloon may be used to dilate several coronary arteries at the same time. Pain is relieved; and patients no longer show evidence on an exercise test that areas of their heart muscle are receiving insufficient blood. Here too, balloon angioplasty is regarded as a possible alternative to bypass surgery.

The idea of balloon angioplasty is attractive. Patients are saved the discomfort of an operation and the inconvenience of long hospital stay. (Discharge after three days is common.) But the balloon procedure is not without risk: much as with coronary artery surgery, there is a mortality of around 1 per cent. Though the tip of the catheter can always be seen on an X-ray screen, it sometimes becomes misplaced. Interference with the coronary artery can provoke potentially fatal abnormalities of heart rhythm; and patients having balloon angioplasty sometimes develop complete blockage of the artery, requiring emergency bypass grafting. So there should always be a team of surgeons nearby who can be called on in an emergency.

Lasers

The other angioplasty technique, not yet out of its research stage, uses laser energy to vaporise plaque. Cleaning up coronary arteries in this way is still largely a laboratory procedure on experimental animals. However, we know that laser light can be directed into the heart using fibre-optics; and that its energy will destroy tissue. In theory, it should be possible to direct the energy precisely enough for diseased tissue to be vaporised, while healthy artery is left intact. This will be easier if researchers can find a wavelength of light that is selectively absorbed by atheroma, and not by normal artery. Lasers are already making important contributions to surgery of the eye in patients with advanced diabetes, where they are used to coagulate blood vessels that threaten sight. They are also successfully used to remove tattoos and skin blemishes. But routine laser surgery on the heart is still some years away.

Home and implanted defibrillation

Many people with a heart attack feel intense chest pain, but do not collapse. However, in around one in three people, the heart is so badly affected by the interruption to its blood supply that the muscle starts to twitch uncontrollably. In this state, called ventricular fibrillation, little if any blood is pumped, the brain is deprived of oxygen and the patient becomes unconscious. Death follows quickly unless resuscitation procedures can be started or normal heart rhythm restored.

In hospital, an emergency team equipped with a defibrillator is never far away. Large paddle electrodes applied to the chest, and a powerful electric shock or two, are usually sufficient to jolt the heart back into normal rhythm and restore the circulation. The problem is that most people who collapse with ventricular fibrillation do so in their own homes. However quickly medical help is sought, and however fast and well-equipped the ambulance that arrives, it is often too late to save the patient's life.

Ideally, people who are clearly at risk of a heart attack should have a portable defibrillator in their own home, for use in emergency by their spouse or whoever else is to hand. Since there is danger in giving a large electric shock to a heart that is not in fibrillation, and since a lay person could not be expected to make the diagnosis, any home defibrillator would have to be capable of confirming fibrillation before it went into action. The device would therefore first have to check the ECG, and be equipped with a sophisticated enough computer to analyse it with very little chance of error. Such devices are now under development.

A variation on the theme of preventing death from sudden abnormalities of heart rhythm following a heart attack is to have anti-arrhythmic drugs more readily available. There is evidence from a recent study in Holland that early administration of lignocaine can halve the chances of ventricular fibrillation in the critical hour or so after a heart attack, and before the patient reaches hospital. One possibility would be to issue all ambulance crews with the drug; another to issue self-injectable supplies to people at highest risk of a heart attack. The dilemma, though, is that probably only half the cases of sudden and severe chest pain are due to a heart attack. We therefore have to be very confident lignocaine does not cause serious adverse effects in patients with non-cardiac problems before we can recommend its use outside proper medical supervision.

As well as people at risk of heart attack, there are those who doctors know are threatened specifically by repeated episodes of ventricular fibrillation. In some of these people, long-term drug therapy does not adequately prevent the problem. This leaves electrical treatment – to reverse any fibrillation that occurs – as an alternative. One possibility is to *implant* a small defibrillator in the patient himself, much as pacemakers have been implanted for years. The device continuously monitors heart rhythm through a pair of electrodes, and delivers a shock through the same electrodes if it detects a life-threatening abnormality. Implantable defibrillators are in use in America, where first reports suggest that they considerably reduce the chances of death from ventricular fibrillation. At the moment, however, their cost (£8,000–10,000) is a deterrent to widespread use.

'Smart' pacemakers

Implantable defibrillators that make a diagnosis before they act are one example of a new generation of 'smart' pacemakers. Abnormalities of heart rhythm other than ventricular fibrillation – though less extreme – may still pose a threat to life, even if only because they cause unpredictable attacks of unconsciousness. Long-term drug treatment for such abnormalities may be ineffective, inconvenient or unwise – if a woman wishes to become pregnant, for example. There is also the worrying fact that all drugs used to treat arrhythmias have the capacity occasionally to induce them.

Sophisticated electronic devices are therefore being devised to detect and reverse many forms of arrhythmia. These pacemakers would lie dormant for most of a patient's life, becoming active only when their microchips recognised a dangerous pattern of electrical activity. Inserting an additional electric shock at a precise point in an abnormal circuit is often sufficient to break it, as are fast bursts of impulses. The most highly developed devices can recognise a variety of unusual patterns of electrical activity, adopt strategies for ending them and adjust their pattern of response until they succeed. They will probably be used increasingly as an alternative to preventive drug therapy.

Artificial and animal hearts

The world's first artificial human heart was implanted by surgeons at Utah University in 1982. One of the carbon valves fractured on the thirteenth day. That was unlucky, but highlights the problem of finding mechanical equivalents as reliable as the human components they seek to replace. There were also difficulties in adjusting the output of the heart, with overuse of antibiotics (which caused problems with the patient's stomach and intestine) and with internal bleeding caused by drugs given in an attempt to prevent the formation of clots. This last problem is a particularly severe test for doctors trying to use a mechanical heart. The interaction between blood and artificial surfaces is well known to produce blood clots, with consequent risk of stroke and damage to other vital organs. As it happened, the first artificial heart patient, Barney Clark, died as a result of strokes and kidney failure after 112 days.

That first implant of a mechanical heart followed twenty years of development, costing $160 million. Yet the patient still had to be connected to an external source of compressed air to power the heart. This meant that mobility and quality of life would have been severely restricted even if the machinery and drug therapy had worked perfectly. In 1984, the same surgeon, William de Vries, implanted another artificial heart in a different hospital, the Humana in Louisville, Kentucky. That patient also died. Rather than being used as a permanent replacement, mechanical hearts are now finding favour as a temporary 'bridging' measure, enabling a patient to survive until a human heart transplant becomes available.

Further research could certainly improve reliability and miniaturise the components in an artificial heart. It could also lead to the development of a power source small enough to be placed inside the patient – if a way could be found of dissipating its heat – and might even replace the natural pulsing action of the heart (necessary because contraction is the only way muscle can work) by some form of rotary pump providing a continuous flow of blood. But the advent of a permanently implantable artificial heart is probably further away than was thought a few years ago.

Efforts at perfecting devices that take heart function over partially and on a temporary basis are probably more worthwhile. Such 'assist' devices have already been successfully implanted. Use of animal hearts for a similar purpose is also a possibility. There are people who see a future in which animals are raised in 'organ farms' to provide spare parts for human surgery. Such a development is feasible, since animals could probably be genetically engineered so that their tissues were not recognised as foreign by our immune systems. This would overcome the problem of organ rejection, which continues to plague transplant surgery despite the development of drugs that reduce our immune response.

Predicting heart attacks

Doctors often have great difficulty in advising patients with heart disease since there is so much uncertainty about what will happen in any invidual case. In George Eliot's novel *Middlemarch*, the doctor is faced with a patient suffering from 'fatty degeneration of the heart', which we now know as angina. 'It is my duty to tell you that death in this disease is often sudden,' says the doctor. 'At the same time, no such result can be predicted. Your condition may be consistent with a tolerably comfortable life for another 15 years or more.' Modern medical and surgical treatment has reduced the chances of sudden death, but the *uncertainty* about outcome for any one patient was much the same in the 1970s as it was in the 1870s when George Eliot wrote. (This example is taken from an essay on the historical background of angina by Dr M. B. Matthews in *Angina Pectoris*, edited by Desmond Julian, Churchill Livingstone, 1977.)

To some extent the position is now changing, thanks to more sophisticated diagnostic techniques which identify the precise site of the obstruction to blood supply. For people who already have symptoms of heart disease, greater knowledge of their exact problem brings the ability to tailor therapy to their particular needs. Revealing the state of the coronary arteries by the injection of X-ray opaque dye (angiography) has shown the way. And we may soon be able to obtain information that is just as precise without exposing patients to the risk involved in inserting a catheter into their hearts.

Nuclear magnetic resonance (NMR) offers promise in this respect. The images now being produced of the heart allow individual coronary arteries to be seen. Allied techniques already measure the flow of blood in larger vessels. If they can be adapted to the finer circulation in the coronary arteries, patients with established disease

can be investigated with less discomfort. With NMR, risk-free mass
screening of large populations also becomes a real possibility.

Among people who have no symptoms, the standard risk factors
such as smoking, weight and diet are notoriously bad at predicting
who will suffer from heart disease. But combination with the exercise ECG (*see* chapter 3) greatly improves their usefulness. Conventional risk factors plus two or more exercise ECG abnormalities
isolates a small group of men (around 1 per cent of those screened)
whose risk of angina, a heart attack or sudden death is increased
33 times. This sort of result (obtained from a ten-year study in
Seattle) begins to make ECG community screening look worthwhile;
and it could be done at far less cost than with NMR.

Lowering cholesterol and reversing atheroma

We already have drugs that lower levels of cholesterol circulating
in the blood. The compounds available at the moment tend to be
inconvenient to take or involve risks that make them unsuitable for
use except by people already in particular danger from heart disease.
Nevertheless, they have proved effective in reducing the incidence
of heart attack and angina, and more palatable drugs with similar
effects are under investigation. (There are more details of results
using existing drugs in chapter 12.)

Whether we will ever have drugs that *remove* atheroma already
present in the arteries is a different question. So far, there appears
to be little prospect.

Measuring quality of life

In many countries, the rapid expansion of opportunities for medical
and surgical therapy places increasing burdens on limited health
budgets. Different forms of treatment compete for scarce resources.
Is coronary artery bypass surgery more valuable than an operation
to replace an arthritic hip? Is long-term drug treatment better used
to prevent stroke in the elderly or to reduce the risk of a second
heart attack in the middle-aged? Curative therapy also competes for
resources with health education aimed at prevention.

The requirement for some objective measure of the costs and
benefits of competing proposals is now generally recognised. So too

is the need to think not just in terms of *quantity* of life – of the extra months or years a patient survives – but of its *quality*. Quality of life is notoriously difficult to measure: but the concept certainly includes freedom from pain, mobility and the ability to enjoy social relationships. Health economists are developing measures which combine these elements and applying them to the outcomes of different forms of treatment. Their studies should enable communities to make difficult decisions about health priorities, as well as helping individual patients choose between alternative courses of treatment.

Chapter Twelve

Can We Avoid Heart Disease?

'Choose your parents carefully' is a distinctly impractical piece of advice on how to avoid heart problems, but it reflects an undoubted fact: there *is* a tendency for coronary artery disease to run in families. People whose parents died young of a heart attack run an increased risk of having one themselves. However, even for those of us with an unfavourable family history, there is nothing inevitable about the outcome. For the majority of the population, there is much that can be done to improve the chances of keeping a healthy heart.

That the heart should eventually wear out with prolonged use is no surprise, but failures of the heart and blood vessels cause half of all deaths in men aged 45–54; and that, by any standards, is young to die – of heart disease or of anything else. At the moment, more than four of every ten premature deaths are cardiovascular in cause. In the USA, more than five million people have symptoms of coronary artery disease, and half a million die from it each year. In Britain, the annual death rate from heart and circulatory disease is 140,000 people under the age of 75.

One thousand heart deaths in the UK are of children with congenital defects of the kind described in chapter 2. Advances in surgery mean that doctors can now save many who would once have died, but congenital malformations of the heart will continue to occur. This is also true of certain faults that develop with the heart's electrical system, and with infections that affect its valves and muscle.

However, the great bulk of heart disease, which is caused by the build-up of fatty deposits along the walls of the coronary arteries, is probably preventable. Most of the rest of this chapter is concerned with the avoidable conditions – angina and heart attack – that are a consequence.

Evidence suggesting heart disease can be prevented

The suddenly increased rate of heart disease

Speaking to the Royal College of Physicians in 1910, William Osler reported that among 2,000 medical cases admitted to London's St Bartholomew's Hospital there were two cases of angina. Later, he wrote that a physician in a large hospital could expect to see one case per year.It was said by a contemporary that the disease affected mostly 'wealthy and commercial folk prone to eat and drink too much'. Many doctors found that only patients in their private practice suffered heart attacks, and routinely recommended ocean cruising as convalescence. In 1926, coronary heart disease accounted for fewer than 1 per cent of deaths in Britain. Now it accounts for 30 per cent.

Looking at time trends in the incidence of disease is notoriously tricky. Expectations change and complaints grow to fill the health services available. There are fashions in diagnosis and in writing death certificates as in everything else; and the changing incidence of one disease can radically affect the perceived impact of another. So distinguishing real differences from apparent ones is difficult.

In Osler's day there were probably many unrecorded cases of angina. People were made invalids by it and stayed at home for 20 years 'with a heart condition' and without expecting a hospital to do anything about it. Undoubtedly, much of the increase in heart disease has occurred because fewer people are dying of other causes, notably infections such as tuberculosis that were rampant under poor socioeconomic conditions and in the pre-antibiotic era. But even when these factors are taken into account, the incidence of heart disease has risen dramatically in a short period of time.

There are three reasons for believing that much coronary heart disease is preventable. The first is that only a few decades ago, no substantial problem existed. Diseases that can emerge so rapidly are not inevitable accompaniments of ageing. They are products of our environment and lifestyle: hazards of modern life, just like road accidents. Having realised this, we can develop strategies to minimise the risk. The encouraging fact is that diseases that suddenly become more common attract attention aimed at identifying

their cause and cure, and potentially can just as quickly be forced
into retreat.

Differences between countries

The second reason for thinking heart disease can be prevented is
that not all countries suffer from it to the same extent. These
geographical differences are very large. Japan, for example, has a
rate of heart disease which is only one-tenth that found in Britain
and the United States. Of course, it could be argued that the
difference lies in the fact that the Japanese are racially distinct, and
so perhaps genetically less susceptible. But we know this is not the
reason because Japanese who emigrate to America soon start to have
increased risk of heart disease, as their style of life adjusts to that
of their host country.

Historical trends and geographical differences are pointers to
preventability. However, the most important reason for optimism
is the demonstration that countries *can* radically reduce heart disease
risk.

Tackling risk factors reduces the disease

North Karelia, the easternmost province of Finland, used to have
the highest rate of coronary heart disease in the world. When this
became known, residents petitioned their government to act. The
government responded, and in ten years the proportion of North
Karelians dying from heart attacks had been reduced by a quarter.
This improvement was achieved both by changes in lifestyle, and
by the increased availability of health screening. Many Finnish
farmers and foresters used to drink six pints of milk a day. Consumption of dairy products has now fallen, and levels of cholesterol
in the blood are down. In the ten years from 1972 to 1982, the
proportion of middle-aged men who smoked fell from 52 to 38 per
cent. Over the same period, the provision of walk-in screening
clinics has improved the medical control of blood pressure.

In New Zealand, where eating of dairy products has declined by
a fifth in the past 20 years, there has been a 5 per cent reduction
overall in plasma cholesterol, and heart disease deaths among middle-aged men are down by 40 per cent. On a national scale, such
figures may seem remote enough to have little impact, but recent
research from Auckland shows more clearly what that means in

practice for a medium-sized city of 180,000 people. Heart disease death rates in 1971 were calculated and extrapolated to 1984. Subtracting the number of deaths that actually occurred showed that 126 lives of men younger than 70 years had been saved. Forty per cent of these lives were thought to have been saved by improved medical facilities, including ambulances specialising in immediate care, and better treatment of blood pressure. But 60 per cent were attributed to changes in smoking and eating habits.

Equally impressive demonstrations of what can be achieved come from Australia and the USA, where heart disease deaths were once far more common than in Britain. Mortality rates plateaued there in the 1960s, and have now fallen by 20 per cent to match those in England and Wales.

Much of the research that linked heart disease with particular risk factors such as smoking was done in Britain. Yet (with the possible exception of Scotland) the UK has been slow to act. 'Analyis breeds paralysis' is the way one community physician has put it. The result is that rates of heart disease have not declined. Among men, the risk seems to have levelled out, and may now be starting to fall. But among women there is evidence still of a slight increase. Compared with 30 years ago, there are now far fewer men who smoke. However, the number of women smoking has risen, which is thought to be the factor responsible.

To some extent the period of inaction is now over. Beginning in 1985, the Health Education Council and the Welsh Office have joined forces to mount an intensive five-year campaign to reduce the incidence of heart disease in Wales. It seeks to emulate the North Karelia project, and the equally successful Stanford Heart Disease Prevention Program in California. If it succeeds in Wales, the campaign will be extended to the rest of the UK.

Can we reduce the risk?

So far we have discussed preventing coronary artery disease as if there were complete agreement on the factors responsible. In fact, there is often considerable dispute, and conclusive evidence is difficult to obtain. Much of our information comes from comparisons between different groups of people at different times. This is often enough to establish an *association* between certain factors and heart disease, but this is not the same as establishing a *cause*. For example, the rise in home ownership in Britain parallels the rise in the incidence of heart disease. However, no one suggests that owning a house causes coronary disease.

Similarly, when rates of heart disease begin to fall, they do so in the context of many changes in the environment and in people's behaviour. Teasing apart the influence of these different factors requires studies that involve many thousands of people and last for decades. Rarely, if ever, can we identify a single change as *the* one relevant to heart disease.

On occasions, ideas suggested by changes in the patterns of disease can be put to genuine test by laboratory experiment. Typically, in the case of heart disease, this involves feeding animals with particular diets. However, the type of coronary disease that occurs so readily in man under 'normal' living conditions has no parallel among free-living animals, and cannot be reproduced exactly even in the laboratory. The relevance of the results that emerge is therefore again arguable.

Even when research enables us to be fairly confident that we have found a cause, there is debate about what to do with the knowledge. Doctors differ as much as any section of the population in their enthusiasm for change. Many, on the evangelical wing, talk of 'the Western way of death' and argue that the 'epidemic' of heart disease can be countered only if whole societies radically alter their eating and leisure habits. Others favour advice directed selectively only at those people who can be identified as at highest risk of heart disease.

These points should be borne in mind when the following sections are read. Ultimately, individuals must make up their own minds about the strength of the evidence and the likely personal benefits and costs of taking it into account. We start with the causes of heart disease that we can be most confident about (though there is room for debate even here) and then move on to those that raise more controversy.

Generally, the risk factors for the first occurrence of heart problems and for their *recurrence* are thought to be similar. So they are probably as relevant in preventing a deterioration in angina or a second heart attack as they are in avoiding heart disease in the first place.

Smoking

Though lung cancer is the condition most dramatically asso
with cigarettes, heart disease caused by smoking kills many more
people. The more cigarettes a person has smoked, the greater the
risk. The increased danger is most apparent early in life, since
younger people tend to show less effect from the other risk factors.
Young smokers may increase their risk of heart attack ten times.
Overall, the effect of smoking is probably to double risk. People
who continue smoking after their first heart attack are significantly
more likely to have a second.

No one is sure of the constituent in cigarette smoke which damages the heart and blood vessels. It could be nicotine. This drug
releases adrenaline and noradrenaline and increases heart rate. Nicotine also affects the behaviour of blood platelets and substances
that cause blood clotting. On the other hand, the prime culprit
could be carbon monoxide gas (which reduces the oxygen-carrying
capacity of the blood), or one of the hundreds of noxious substances
not yet investigated. Pipe and cigar smokers absorb nicotine through
the lining of the mouth, even when they do not inhale; yet they do
not seem to have increased risk of heart disease. This is some
evidence suggesting nicotine is not responsible. But the position is
still unclear.

The good news is that once someone gives up cigarettes, their
risk of heart attack starts to decrease almost immediately. So too
does the severity of any continuing symptoms. Switching to milder,
low-tar cigarettes is not very helpful since smokers compensate for
the reduced availability of nicotine by smoking more frequently and
inhaling more.

Blood pressure

High blood pressure (hypertension) leads to greater wear and tear
on the entire system of blood vessels. In both men and women it
roughly doubles the risk of heart attack and stroke. Even moderately
raised levels appreciably increase the risks of these two events. In
the most severe cases, high blood pressure may also damage the
kidneys and enlarge the left ventricle of the heart, decreasing the
efficiency with which it pumps and increasing the risk of heart
failure.

In more than 90 per cent of people who have hypertension there is no identifiable cause. However, drug treatment is usually effective at lowering blood pressure. The most frequently used drugs are beta-blockers and diuretics. A vasodilator, an ACE inhibitor or an agent specifically developed for blood pressure control may also be prescribed. All of these drugs are described in chapter 13.

Blood pressure is usually given as two values: the first refers to the pressure in the arteries when the heart contracts (systolic) and the second to the lower pressure when the heart relaxes (diastolic). Like atmospheric pressure, blood pressure is measured in millimetres of mercury (which is abbreviated to mmHg).

Typical readings for the two pressures are 120 and 80 – often expressed as 120/80 – though a range of pressures either side of these points would also be considered normal. Deciding the exact definition of 'high' is therefore difficult. Just as with weight and height, a few people are found at the low and high extremes, but the great majority lie somewhere not far above or below the average. Another problem is that blood pressures can vary considerably through the day, and may be higher because a patient is anxious about having it measured than it otherwise would be. This means that blood pressure should be taken on several occasions, ideally at different times of day, and in as relaxed an atmosphere as possible.

Often, high blood pressure produces no symptoms. Many people who have serious hypertension are therefore entirely unaware of the fact. This means that regular blood pressure checks (every two or three years) are important. Anyone offered the chance of blood pressure screening should take it. Women are just as likely to be affected as men.

A diastolic pressure in middle age which is consistently over 110 is usually accepted as requiring treatment. Below this point is a grey area, but it would be reasonable to class a diastolic pressure greater than 90 as mildly hypertensive. A systolic pressure greater than 180 should be treated, and some doctors would argue hypertension starts with a systolic level of 160 or lower.

If high blood pressure is taken as anything greater than 160 mm systolic or 100 mm diastolic, then perhaps nine million people in the UK have hypertension. That includes one in three of all people who reach the age of 70. However, substantial numbers are far younger; and their presence is significant. Someone aged 40 with hypertension is five times more likely to die early than someone of the same age with a normal blood pressure.

Should mild hypertension be treated?

There is as much debate about control of mildly raised blood pressure as about any aspect of heart disease prevention. It is clear that if blood pressure is well above normal, taking drugs to lower it will reduce the chances of heart attack and stroke. But if blood pressure is only a little raised (say between 90 and 100 mm diastolic), medical treatment may not be worthwhile. We can now say this with some certainty because the results of two ten-year studies of anti-hypertensive drugs were published in 1985. Each study compared large groups of patients taking drugs to control blood pressure with similar groups who took only dummy, placebo tablets.

Among those taking drugs, there were fewer cases of stroke, and (among the over 60s) fewer cases also of fatal heart attack. We can be confident from the statistics that these differences between treated and untreated patients are not the product of chance. For example, people taking anti-hypertensive drugs were only *half* as likely to have a stroke.

That sounds an impressive difference; and among people older than 60 it may be a genuinely useful reduction. However, for people who are under 60 and have mild hypertension, the real benefit is little, since the risk of stroke is tiny even among those who receive no drugs. The results of the Medical Research Council trial in the UK show that doctors would have to treat 850 people with mild hypertension for a year before they could say with confidence that a single stroke had been prevented. In other words, in the case of any *particular* middle-aged person with mild hypertension, taking a drug is unlikely to make very much difference. The chance of being among the 849 who would not suffer anyway is far greater than of being the one person saved by drugs from a stroke.

Of course, if there were no side-effects of medication, there would be no argument against taking it and being on the safe side. But there *are* potential side-effects: costs as well as benefits. Taking drugs such as beta-blockers long-term can make a person feel unwell, and men may experience impotence. Use of diuretics (which increase urine production) may deplete the body of essential supplies of potassium. And both kinds of drugs have been associated with changes in the levels of fats in the blood that may actually work against the health of the heart. (Incidentally, large studies suggest that diuretics and beta-blockers are similarly effective in the control of blood pressure.)

These considerations are swinging the pendulum against drug treatment of *mild* hypertension. But they do not mean that nothing should be done. Drinking less alcohol and losing weight have no side-effects, and also decrease blood pressure. In addition, reducing consumption of salt and learning techniques of relaxation may be helpful.

Excess weight

Obesity is linked to a higher risk of heart disease. Unnecessary deposits of fat impose extra strain on the heart which has to supply it with blood as well as carry the increased weight around. In Western countries, one in three adults is regarded as overweight, and one in 20 is obese. Excess weight increases with age, but should be tackled young, since fat children and adolescents tend to become fat adults.

Excess weight seems to increase the overall risk of death, but may be particularly damaging to people who have diabetes or a family history of cardiovascular disease. However, the direct contribution made by excess weight is difficult to establish since being fat is clearly associated with high blood pressure, and with particular, potentially harmful eating habits. Smokers weigh less on average than non-smokers, but the risks of continuing to smoke are greater than the risks of putting on a few pounds in weight.

Figures 12.1 and 12.2 give the average weights, the acceptable ranges and the lower limits of obesity, according to height, for men and women, respectively. The figures are taken from the report by the UK National Advisory Committee on Nutrition Education, published by the Health Education Council, London, 1983. In turn, they are based on recommendations made by the Fogarty Conference in the USA and the Royal College of Physicians, London.

Cholesterol

Cholesterol is a substance found in animal fats. Its notoriety arises from the belief that too much cholesterol in our diet leads to the development of atheroma deposits in our arteries and so to coronary heart disease; but whether it does so in any straightforward way is

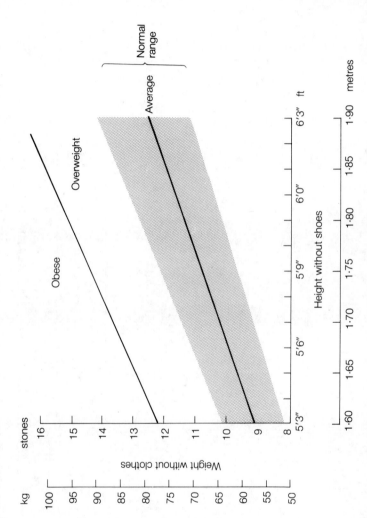

Figure 12.1 Acceptable weight ranges and the border of obesity: men.

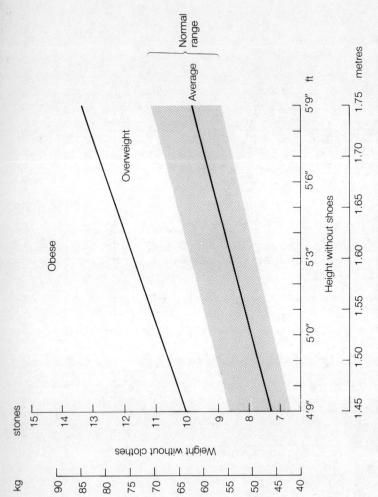

Figure 12.2 Acceptable weight ranges and the borders of obesity: women.

a vexed question. The consensus of scientific opinion seems to be that cholesterol is at least partly to blame.

We must admit that there is no *proof* that lowering cholesterol levels will do us good. However, in the light of the evidence available, it would be prudent to reduce our intake of red meat, dairy products and eggs, since these are the major dietary sources of cholesterol. For most people, though, there is no need to be obsessive about this aspect of diet.

Fats in foods and fats in blood are not necessarily the same thing. The amount and type of fat in our diet usually has some effect on the fat in our blood, but there would be fats in blood even if we ate none at all. The two most important substances making up blood fats (or, to use the medical term, blood *lipids*) are cholesterol and triglycerides. The heart disease debate has centered on cholesterol, and it is on this substance that we concentrate.

Far from being a poison, cholesterol is an essential part of all cells. Two-thirds of the 150 grams that we contain is made by our own bodies. However, the food we eat is also a source of cholesterol, and several facts suggest these additional amounts are the fundamental cause of coronary heart disease.

Evidence that cholesterol causes heart disease

First, much of the fatty deposit that collects along the walls of our arteries, and which in some cases completely blocks them, is cholesterol. Secondly, people who have a genetic defect which means that the body cannot properly deal with cholesterol have high levels of the substance in their blood and develop coronary heart disease at a young age. If patients with these inherited problems are given a drug that lowers cholesterol level, fewer of them develop heart disease. Thirdly, it is possible to produce fatty deposits along the arteries of animals by feeding them on a diet which is rich in cholesterol, though the form of disease produced by experiments in animals is not the same as that occurring naturally in ourselves.

Finally, there is evidence from studies we have mentioned that compare the rates of heart disease in different countries. This research shows a reasonably clear association between the amount of cholesterol in the typical diet, the average levels of cholesterol circulating in people's blood and the risk of death from heart disease. For example, during 1972 in East Finland (where there was large consumption of meat and dairy products and the worst heart disease record in the world at that time) there were high levels of blood cholesterol: an average of 280 milligrams in every 100 millilitres of blood. In Japan, with only one-tenth of the heart disease and a largely rice and fish diet, the cholesterol level was less than 180 milligrams.

Evidence that the association between high blood cholesterol levels and heart disease is cause and effect – and not simply coincidental – comes from the results of *intervention* studies. Here, health authorities step in to persuade a population to lower its intake of cholesterol, and then assess the results. The usual finding is that less cholesterol in the diet leads to less cholesterol in the blood, and to lower rates of heart disease. In East Finland, for example, blood cholesterol levels in men fell from 276 milligrams to 246. Over the same period, the number of deaths from heart disease was declining by over 3 per cent each year.

Using these sources of evidence, government health agencies have advised us to reduce the amount of cholesterol in our diet. In the UK, the Health Education Council recommends that we should obtain only 30 per cent of our total energy intake from fats. At the moment – even when we include the energy found in alcohol – we obtain 38 per cent of our calories from fat. Eating fewer dairy products and less red meat would cut our fat consumption, while increasing the amount of fish and fowl maintained sources of animal protein. At the same time, reducing sugar intake would do much to counter our undoubted tendency towards overweight. (Sugar is 'empty' calories: it provides energy but has no other nutritional value.) Increases in fibre-rich cereals, pulses, fruit and vegetables would help shift our diet towards greater health for the heart.

The other side of the story

The changes in diet that health authorities suggest, and the reasons for their suggestions, have been considered. However, when looked at in greater detail, the argument becomes more complex.

First, the type of fat found in the arteries of patients who have severe heart disease is not the same as that in the diet. And earlier fatty deposits along the wall of the artery that were once thought to be the first stage of the disease – and which do contain cholesterol – do not develop in any straightforward way into the kind of deposits that cause the real problems.

It is true that people who have inherited defects of cholesterol metabolism have high levels of cholesterol in their blood and, if not treated, are likely to die early from heart disease. But the levels of cholesterol that are clearly harmful in these inherited conditions are very high indeed. We cannot infer from this evidence that *moderate* levels of cholesterol do any damage at all. An analogy can be drawn with diabetes. People whose bodies cannot handle sugar in the usual way must avoid it. However, for those with normal metabolism sugar poses no threat (except indirectly via overweight and tooth decay).

Next, there are important exceptions to the overall association between blood cholesterol levels, diet and disease. Some regions have a high intake of fat and yet relatively low rates of heart attack. Western Finland, for example, eats almost as much fat as the east of the country, and yet has only one-third of the mortality from heart disease.

We vary greatly in the amount of cholesterol in our diets. Yet the differences between us in blood cholesterol are relatively small. Evidence from experiments suggests that if you increase the amount of cholesterol in food (by adding extra eggs to the diet, for example), the body either does not absorb the additional cholesterol or responds by producing less cholesterol itself.

Even if large amounts of cholesterol in the diet translate into large amounts in the blood, the relationship with heart disease is not straightforward. Some studies show that high levels of blood cholesterol predict the occurrence of heart disease several years later. But in Israel, for example, people with moderately raised levels of blood cholesterol suffer no more heart attacks than those with low blood cholesterol levels.

Finally, not all health education projects have as much impact as the Finnish experience in North Karelia suggests. In particular, a major initiative in the United States (called MR FIT, the Multiple Risk Factor Intervention Trial) recently proved largely a failure, for all the $120 million spent on it. There was some reduction in cholesterol intake among the group of men who were given intensive advice on changing their lifestyle, though it was less than had been hoped. This raises questions about the feasibility of persuading large numbers of people to change the way they live. More important, there was no appreciable decrease in the number of people who died from heart attacks. This suggested that even if risk factors were reduced, people might not be any better off.

So far, we have discussed the link with heart disease in terms simply of cholesterol. However, cholesterol itself does not seem to be the problem, but rather the way cholesterol is carried in the blood. On its own, cholesterol (like other lipids) would not dissolve. To be transported, it therefore has to be attached to other substances (mostly proteins) to form tiny particles. These particles, called lipoproteins, come in several forms, which differ in density. Low density lipoprotein (LDL) is thought to carry cholesterol *into* the arterial wall where it is deposited. For this reason, it is thought to be bad to have large quantities of low density lipoproteins circulating in the blood. High density lipoproteins (HDL), on the other hand, take cholesterol *away* from the artery wall. Finding high levels of HDL in the blood is therefore a good sign.

So, measuring the level of total cholesterol in the blood is not enough. We need to know the way it is distributed between the HDL and LDL forms. This has been realised only recently, and it is possible that the conflicting evidence we have on cholesterol results from our earlier failure to take this into account.

To add to the uncertainty, we are now finding out about factors that seem to predict the risk of heart disease better than cholesterol. These new predictors are chemicals in the blood that control the rate at which it coagulates and forms clots. One important substance appears to be fibrinogen. People who have high levels of fibrinogen in their blood are more likely to die of coronary heart disease.

It is known that fibrin – which is formed from fibrinogen – is part of the structure of fatty deposits in the artery wall (*see* chapter 2). It is also closely involved in the formation of clots which may block arteries that have already become narrowed, precipitating a heart attack. (In extreme circumstances, the coagulability of the blood may be sufficiently abnormal for clots to form and block even those arteries that are of normal diameter.) There is increasing evidence that drugs which decrease coagulation effectively reduce the chances of a second heart attack in people who have already had one (*see* chapter 4). An intriguing twist to the coagulation story is that the behaviour of clotting factors may depend on diet, and especially on fat intake. So following this different lead may bring us full circle back to diet after all.

Taken together, the evidence that diet is somehow involved in coronary heart disease seems pretty impressive. But there are distinguished doctors and scientists who have genuine doubts about almost every point. That is the reason for caution in giving strict dietary advice in the absence of specific abnormalities in the way our bodies handle cholesterol.

Exercise

Exercise is generally considered beneficial for the heart and circulation. As with any muscle, the heart may work better for being fit; and it is possible that exercise leads to a widening of the crucial coronary arteries. But it is an important fact that heart disease is now more common among manual workers, who are physically active in their jobs, than among professional people, who tend to be sedentary. Once the position was quite the reverse. This suggests that being physically active may not itself be enough to protect against heart disease.

There is undoubtedly an association between lower rates of heart attack and leisure-time exercise. Studies have suggested that to be of benefit, the exercise must be regular (three or more times per week for half an hour or so) and sufficiently strenuous to cause sweating and some breathlessness. However, people who take this amount of exercise tend also to be non-smokers who are not overweight and who pay attention to their diet. It is therefore difficult to disentangle any effect of exercise from the influence of these other, related factors.

Moderate exercise, with a doctor's advice, can play an important part in physical and psychological rehabilitation after a heart attack. This topic is covered in chapter 5.

Stress and personality

Personality seems to play a part in coronary heart disease. The evidence comes from the same kind of long-term, follow-up studies (such as at Framingham) that reveal the other risk factors. The strongest evidence is that people who have competitive, driving, hostile personalities are more prone to angina and heart attacks than those who are more easy-going. The coronary-prone personality is called 'Type A'. It is not clear exactly how personality and heart disease are linked, but people with Type A personality appear to differ in their biochemical and behavioural response to stress.

Stress is believed to increase the level of cholesterol that circulates in our bloodstream. It may therefore be linked to heart disease through the whole complicated cholesterol story. Stress also increases the levels of other substances, notably the hormones adrenaline and noradrenaline. These biochemical responses exist to gear us for physical exertion – either fight or flight. In other aspects of the response, blood is diverted from outlying parts of the body to its centre, our heart rate and blood pressure rise, and the level of fuels that power the muscles is increased. All of these changes are clearly useful when we really may have to run for our lives or defend ourselves physically. But they are of doubtful value if the constraints of civilisation preclude either course of action; and there is a suspicion that a stress response induced time after time without being properly 'discharged' has destructive effects on the heart and circulation.

It is possible that training in techniques of relaxation may reduce the likelihood of a second heart attack, and that simple breathing exercises and strategies for coping with stress decrease the chances of people at risk developing angina and other signs of coronary artery disease. Such effects may be direct, or appear as the result of alterations in other risk factors. In some studies, relaxation reduces blood pressure and cigarette consumption, for example.

Alcohol

Some studies have found that light drinkers (one or two drinks per day) have less heart disease than those who do not drink at all: a finding that has been taken as evidence for the popular belief that a little alcohol is 'good for the circulation'. Since alcohol dilates blood vessels, it may marginally relieve the work of the heart. However, there are doubts about the way information on drinking has been collected in these studies, and the relationship has not been confirmed.

Heavy drinking, on the other and, is assuredly *bad* – for the heart as well as for the liver, stomach and brain. Excessive alcohol consumption increases blood pressure, makes hypertension more difficult to treat, exaggerates the tendency to overweight, and seems to produce abnormalities in the pattern of blood lipids.

Diabetes

Though we turn to it at this late stage in our account of risk factors, since relatively few people are affected, diabetes undoubtedly increases the likelihood of coronary heart disease. Lack of insulin means that glucose stays in the blood and is not properly transferred into the body's cells, where it acts as their major source of energy. They therefore work less efficiently. In diabetes, the metabolism of blood fats as well as blood sugar is abnormal.

The precise reasons are still unknown, but these biochemical abnormalities combine to encourage the development of atheroma in the arteries. Being a diabetic also seems to increase the seriousness of the consequences. Diabetics who have a heart attack are at greater risk of developing heart failure and are less likely to recover. This may be because diabetes itself also produces gradual, long-term damage to the heart muscle.

Soft water

A slightly higher risk of heart attack in areas of the country with a soft water supply is a surprising, intriguing and fairly consistent finding of studies that map the incidence of heart disease. Minerals in the water make it hard, so one or other of them may be having a mildly protective effect.

Chapter Thirteen

Drugs Used to Treat Heart Disease

Heart disease is treated using more than 120 different drugs, which can be divided into categories according to their broad chemical composition and their major uses. Table 13.1 shows nine major drug groups and five heart conditions (plus high blood pressure) for which they may be used. This is only a very rough guide, but it clearly shows two things. First, the same type of drug can be taken for a range of reasons; secondly, the same problem can be treated using a variety of different types of drug, alone or in combination with each other. Doctors therefore have great choice in the drugs they prescribe, and can tune therapy to the individual needs of a particular patient.

Though the latest drugs can only be made by the company that discovered them, many older agents are now marketed by several manufacturers, each using their own brand name. Doctors, especially those in general practice, often prescribe drugs by brand, rather than by general, 'approved' chemical name. It may therefore be difficult to track down a particular product. A book like this cannot provide an exhaustive list of all brand names, nor even of all the chemical entities involved, many of which are quite similar. But in this section we try to cover all major drugs, and refer to the most common of their brand names.

Information on drugs is also found in the chapters dealing with particular heart conditions. Drugs that can only be given by injection are mentioned there, and generally do not appear in this section.

In contrast to the position in general practice, drugs given in hospital are usually dispensed by their approved name. Someone leaving hospital and continuing to have drugs prescribed by their family doctor may therefore think their medication has been

Table 13.1 Heart conditions and the main types of drug that may be used to treat them

	Angina	After a heart attack	Heart failure	Abnormal heart rhythms	High blood pressure	Heart valve disease
Beta-blockers	√	(√)	–	(√)	√	–
Diuretics	–	–	√	–	√	(√)
Nitrates	√	–	√	–	–	–
Calcium antagonists	√	–	–	√	√	–
Other vasodilators	–	–	√	–	√	–
ACE inhibitors	–	–	√	–	√	–
Digitalis drugs	–	(√)	–	√	–	(√)
Anti-platelet drugs	(√)	(√)	–	–	–	√
Anti-coagulant drugs	–	–	–	(√)	–	√

changed when it has not. We should also be aware that exactly the same drug, when marketed by different companies, can appear in entirely different shapes, sizes and colours of tablet. So a change in appearance does not necessarily mean a change in drug.

Anyone who is in doubt about what they are taking, or why, should ask. Doctors will be pleased to explain. Community pharmacists (retail chemists) are also available to discuss the drugs they dispense. The basic information used here is taken largely from the *British National Formulary*, the handbook used by doctors and pharmacists when prescribing and dispensing drugs.

In preparing the tables that follow we have included a column showing side-effects. Most of them are infrequent, and usually represent a discomfort rather than a serious threat; but a doctor should be consulted if there is any doubt about their importance. Brand names of drugs begin with a capital letter; general, approved names of drugs do not.

Beta-blockers

Beta-blockers are the closest we have to a cardiac cure-all. They play a part in lowering blood pressure, controlling angina, reducing the chances of a second heart attack and also on occasions preventing abnormalities of heart rhythm. Their versatility does not stop there, since beta-blockers are also used to reduce anxiety, prevent migraine and treat overactivity of the thyroid gland. Concert performers (especially violinists) and snooker players have taken them to reduce tremor, and they are sometimes prescribed for examination nerves.

Since their discovery twenty years ago, beta-blockers have transformed the treatment of heart disease and high blood pressure. The family of drugs derives its name from the fact that it blocks the effects of the body's 'fight or flight' hormones (adrenaline and noradrenaline). Beta-blockers do this by occupying the places on cells (called receptors) where the hormones normally act. The analogy is with a lock and key. Beta-blocker drugs fit the receptor 'keyholes' normally used by the body's hormones, obstructing access to them.

The usual effects of adrenaline and noradrenaline are to increase heart rate, make the cardiac muscle contract more forcefully and constrict blood vessels. By preventing these effects, beta-blockers reduce the oxygen demands of the heart, helping to avoid the pain of angina and enabling people with the condition to tolerate m‿ exercise.

Beta-blockers also gradually reduce blood pressure (taking between two days and two weeks to achieve their effect), though the precise way they do so is still unclear. Where the blood pressure problem is mild, beta-blockers will usually control it. They will often be the first drug tried, with a thiazide (*see* the section on diuretics below) added if necessary. Hypertension is Britain's most diagnosed disease, accounting for 5 per cent of all conditions treated by general practitioners and 10 per cent of all prescriptions.

Recent evidence suggests that certain beta-blockers reduce the risk of death over the few days after a heart attack. The drugs (atenolol or metoprolol) have to be given intravenously within a few hours and then by tablet over the next week. The possible long-term benefits of taking beta-blockers after a heart attack are considered in chapter 5 (*see* p. 73).

With a class of drugs as useful and profitable as the beta-blockers, most pharmaceutical companies have been encouraged to produce their own versions. Once the legal protection afforded the discoverers has expired, any company is free to bring out its own brand of the identical chemical. Manufacturers have also produced a confusing array of 'me-too' drugs, in which a few molecules have been juggled around to produce a chemical which is just different enough from the original to escape legal protection. The result is a confusing array of drugs (table 13.2), though many of them will be familiar, and some brands have achieved the status almost of household names.

The proliferation of beta-blockers should not be viewed too cynically, however. Although similar in their main effects, there *are* some differences in the way they act. There may therefore be drugs which are particularly suited to an individual or especially appropriate to a given complaint. Oxprenolol, pindolol and acebutolol seem to control blood pressure without slowing the heart as much as other beta-blockers. For someone with high blood pressure alone they are therefore an advantage; but when hypertension is combined with angina, for example, the extra reduction of heart rate found with other beta-blockers may be useful. People taking oxprenolol, pindolol and acebutolol also tend to complain less of cold fingers and feet.

Atenolol, nadolol and sotalol are more water- than fat-soluble, and so are less likely to cross the 'blood-brain' barrier and cause

Table 13.2 Beta-blocker drugs: for high blood pressure, angina, arrhythmias and heart attack

Approved names	Brand names	Conditions treated	Possible side-effects
propranolol	Inderal, Angilol, Apsolol, Bedranol, Berkolol, Sloprolol	high blood pressure; angina; abnormal heart rhythm; (perhaps preventing second heart attack)	slow heart rate; cold hands and feet; gastro-intestinal upset; difficulty in breathing (airway constriction); heart failure, nightmares; impotence
sotalol	Beta-Cardone, Sotacor		
timolol	Betim, Blocadren		
acebutalol[a]	Sectral		
atenolol[a]	Tenormin	high blood pressure; angina; abnormal heart rhythm; (perhaps protecting against the effects of a heart attack)	as above
metoprolol[a]	Betaloc, Lopresor		
nadolol	Corgard		
oxprenolol	Trasicor, Apsolox, Laracor, Slow-Pren		
pindolol	Visken	high blood pressure, angina	as above
betaxolol	Kerlone		as above
labetalol	Trandate	high blood pressure	low blood pressure; tiredness; rash
penbutolol	—		as above

The following brands combine a beta-blocker with a thiazide diuretic: Co-Betaloc, Corgaretic, Inderetic, Inderex, Lopresoretic, Moducren, Prestim, Secadrex, Sotazide, Tenoret(ic), Tolerzide, Trasidrex, Viskaldix. Spiroprop combines a beta-blocker with the diuretic spironolactone and Lasipressin with frusemide.

[a] These drugs may be less likely than the others to bring on asthma.

symptoms such as nightmares and insomnia. Another source of difference within the beta-blocker family is in their effects on the lungs. Cells lining the large airways of the lung contain receptors similar to those found in blood vessel walls. But here the effect of beta-blockers may be one of constriction, bringing on asthma in sensitive individuals. This effect is likely to be least with metoprolol, atenolol, acebutolol and labetalol.

Various rather general complaints are laid at the door of beta-blockers. These include tiredness and weakness of the muscles, and impotence. Beta-blockers are not usually suitable for someone who has experienced problems of heart failure.

Diuretics

Diuretics, often called 'water pills' are a large group of drugs (table 13.3) which remove fluid from the body by increasing the amount of salt (sodium) excreted in the urine. In getting rid of salt, the kidneys excrete water too, reducing the amount of fluid in the body and so lowering blood pressure. Diuretics are therefore frequently part of the treatment for high blood pressure, indeed, they may be the only drug, especially in the elderly. To reduce sleep disturbance from the need to urinate, diuretics are often taken early in the day.

The group of diuretics known as thiazides will generally be the first used to control blood pressure, followed by loop diuretics, which have an effect two or three times more powerful. (Loop diuretics get their name because they affect the looped portions of the kidneys' urine-collecting tubules.) Many combinations of diuretics are possible. They may also be combined with other classes of drug such as the vasodilators.

As fluid accumulation (oedema) occurs when the heart is not maintaining an effective circulation, higher doses and the more powerful diuretic drugs also provide valuable relief from the symptoms of heart failure.

Some (but not all) diuretics increase the amount of potassium lost from the body. Since this substance is vital to our healthy functioning, potassium levels may need to be measured in a blood sample and possibly topped up using a supplement. There are also good supplies of potassium in certain foods, such as fresh raw vegetables and fruit. Drugs which have a 'K' added to their trade name already have potassium added.

Table 13.3 Diuretic drugs: for high blood pressure and heart failure

Type of diuretic	Approved names	Brand names	Overall effects	Possible side-effects
thiazides (1)	e.g. bendrofluazide	Aprinox, Berkozide, Centyl, Neo Na-Clex, Urizide	low doses reduce blood pressure; higher doses relieve oedema; gradual onset of effect	deplete body of potassium; raise blood sugar and cholesterol; rashes; impotence; dehydration
	chlorthalidone	Hygroton		
	hydrochlorthiazide	Esidrex, Hydro-Saluric		
'loop diuretics' (2)	frusemide	Lasix, Aluzine, Diuresal, Dryptal, Frusetic, Frusid	faster-acting and more powerful diuretics, used mostly to relieve fluid accumulation in heart failure	loss of potassium; too great a fall in blood pressure; rashes; dehydration
	bumetanide	Burinex		
	ethacrynic acid	Edecrin		
potassium-sparing diuretics (3)	amiloride	Midamor	relatively weak diuretic effect; cause body to *retain* potassium	rashes, mental confusion
	triamterene	Dytac		rashes, gastro-intestinal disturbance
aldosterone antagonists (4)	spironolactone	Aldactone, Diatensec Laractone, Spiretic, Spiroctan, Spirolone	weak action, but extends effect of drugs above	gastro-intestinal disturbance; painful breast enlargement (men and women)

Many tablets are combinations of the above drugs. These include Aldactide (1 combined with 4), Amilco (1,3), Dyazide (1,3), Dytide (1,3), Frumil (2,3), Frusene (2,3), Kalspare (1,3), Lasilactone (2,4), Moduret(ic) (1,3), Synuretic (1,3). Kalten is a thiazide plus a potassium-sparing diuretic plus a beta blocker. See the section on beta-blockers for diuretic/beta-blocker combinations. Other preparations combine the above with a potassium supplement, often signified by the addition of 'K' to the brand name. Additional supplemented diuretics include Brinaldix K (1), Centyl K (1), Diumide K (2), Lasikal (2), Navidrex K (1).

Nitrates

The simple procedure of dissolving a small tablet under the tongue has provided effective relief from pain for several generations of angina sufferers. The drug responsible – glyceryl trinitrate or GTN – works in two ways. Direct expansion of the coronary arteries increases the *supply* of blood to oxygen-deprived muscle. At the same time, the work of the heart is reduced (and its *demand* for fuel therefore decreased) because the drug dilates the body's veins, so slowing the return of blood to the heart. The one major disadvantage of trinitrate is that the drug-induced expansion of blood vessels may lead to a throbbing headache.

The under-the-tongue tablet is the traditional way of taking trinitrate, though it is also available as an aerosol (sprayed into the mouth) and as a pill that is slowly dissolved between the gum and lip. Used before exercise, all three methods of taking the drug effectively prevent the onset of angina; and attacks that have not been foreseen can usually be cured within a few minutes. Therapy is therefore convenient and quickly effective. But trinitrate delivered in these ways does not provide long-term control of angina.

Drug companies have therefore tried to devise ways of giving the drug slowly over a long period. Slow absorption can be obtained by using trinitrate ointment smeared on the skin and from sticky plasters impregnated with the drug (table 13.4). Using either paste or plaster may provide effective long-term relief, especially by preventing angina attacks at night. There are also longer-acting chemicals with similar effects to trinitrate. Isosorbide dinitrate is one example. In small doses, this drug can be used under the tongue; in larger doses it is swallowed and absorbed like most tablets from the stomach and intestine. Some slow-release forms are taken only once a day; others need to be taken more frequently.

The range of chemicals now available and the variety of different ways in which they can be taken provide fertile ground for misunderstanding. Clear instructions on how to use them should be given with each preparation. Trinitrate tablets lose their effectiveness with time, and must be stored in the glass container they are supplied in. Tablets older than eight weeks should be thrown away.

Many patients with angina will find nitrates on their own provide satisfactory therapy. Others, with angina that occurs frequently and

Table 13.4 Nitrates: drugs used to dilate blood vessels in treating angina

Approved names	Preparations/brand names	Possible side-effects
glyceryl trinitrate	tablets: GTN, Natirose, Nitrocontin, Suscard Buccal, Sustac spray: Coro-Nitro, Nitrolingual ointment: Percutol plasters: Transiderm-Nitro	
isosorbide dinitrate	Cedocard (Retard), Isoket (Retard), Isordil, Soni-Slo, Sorbichew, Sorbid, Sorbitrate, Vascardin	throbbing headache, dizziness, flushing, low blood pressure on standing
isosorbide mononitrate	Elantan, Ismo, Monit, Mono-Cedocard	
pentaerythritol tetranitrate	Mycardol, Peritrate	

All preparations are in tablet form unless otherwise specified. But some tablets are dissolved in the mouth while others are swallowed. Read instructions carefully.

in a way unrelated to exercise, will probably need to take other drugs, such as a beta-blocker or clacium antagonist.

Calcium antagonists

The action of calcium within heart muscle cells plays a crucial part in controlling their activity. Drugs that interfere with its effects therefore provide another way of treating heart conditions. Two problems in particular – abnormal heart rhythms and angina – can be effectively controlled using chemicals called calcium antagonists or calcium channel blockers. Calcium blockers may be especially helpful where angina is due not to narrowing of the coronary arteries by atheroma deposited along the blood vessel but to muscular clenching (spasm) of the artery walls.

Nifedipine (Adalat) expands blood vessels in the body and the coronary arteries of the heart and is therefore useful in treating high blood pressure as well as angina. Side-effects include flushing and headache.

Verapamil (Cordilox) is a calcium blocker taken particularly for arrhythmias, as well as for angina. Nausea, vomiting and constipation are possible side-effects. There is also a small risk of a sudden, severe fall in blood pressure and heart rate. Diltiazem (Tildiem) is used primarily to prevent angina. Existing calcium blocker drugs tend to reduce the force with which the heart muscle contracts. This means that they are not advisable in patients with symptoms of heart failure. However, new drugs under development will probably overcome this problem.

Other drugs used to treat high blood pressure

Prazosin (Hypovase) rapidly reduces blood pressure (and may do so too much). But it is used to treat hypertension, and also to expand the blood vessels and so reduce the workload of the failing heart. Phenoxybenzamine (Dibenyline) and indoramin (Baratol) are also effective drugs and, despite their side-effects, may be useful where other drug treatment of high blood pressure has not controlled the problem. The same is true of guanethidine (Ismelin) and debrisoquine (Declinax).

Several drugs control high blood pressure through their actions on the brain. They include methyldopa (Aldomet, Dopamet, Hydromet, Medomet), which may cause depression, drowsiness, diarrhoea and blood and skin disorders in large doses but is regarded as useful in small doses. Unlike beta-blockers, it is safe for people with asthma and heart failure. Clonidine (Catapres) may also cause depression and tiredness. Reserpine and rauwolfia drugs (Rautrax and Serpasil) are little used in Britain, but are more common elsewhere. They too can lead to severe depression.

ACE inhibitors

The venom of a South American pit viper proved the starting point for the development of a completely new class of drugs which is already being successfully used to treat high blood pressure and heart failure. Briefly, the drugs work by blocking an enzyme that converts an inactive protein in the body into one which powerfully constricts blood vessels. (The 'ACE' part of the name stands for angiotensin converting enzyme.) Constricting blood vessels increases the pressure within them; so preventing the constriction effectively reduces blood pressure.

At the moment, only two such drugs are available (though there are soon likely to be many more). They are captopril (Acepril and Capoten) and enalapril (Innovace). Both effectively reduce blood pressure, working about as well on their own as one of the thiazide diuretic drugs. Combined with a thiazide, ACE inhibitors lead to a further fall in blood pressure, and may have the additional helpful action of countering some of the diuretic's side-effects. Many patients switched from other medication to ACE inhibitor drugs say they feel better for it. Skin rashes and abnormal taste sensations are occasional side-effects. More serious complications occur but are rare if the dose is kept low.

ACE inhibitors are being used in people with heart failure, since dilating the arteries is one way of helping the heart. The initial fall in blood pressure may be severe, and for this reason the drugs are often first tried in hospital.

Digitalis drugs

Digitalis drugs are used in heart failure and certain abnormal heart rhythms, especially atrial fibrillation (*see* chapters 7 and 9). Their approved names include digoxin, digitoxin, lanatoside, medigoxin, ouabain. Brand names are the same as the chemical names, plus Lanoxin, Digitaline, Cedilanid, Lanitop. Possible side-effects are loss of appetite, nausea, vomiting, diarrhoea and abnormal heart rhythms.

Cardiac physicians recently celebrated the bicentenary of the publication of the *Account of the Foxglove* by a Birmingham doctor, William Withering, in 1785. Two hundred years after Withering first noticed that extracts of this plant had a beneficial stimulant effect on the heart, digitalis (named after the foxglove's botanical name *Digitalis purpurea*) is still the basis of one of the most important drug groups used to treat heart failure. Digoxin is a standardised preparation of the drug; digitoxin and the other chemicals mentioned above are closely related. The digitalis drugs also go by the name 'cardiac glycosides'.

In certain patients, though possibly not in all, digoxin improves the efficiency with which the heart pumps blood, by raising supplies of calcium within the heart muscle cells. When used to control abnormalities of heart rhythm (specifically atrial fibrillation) the digitalis drugs work by slowing the rate of conduction through the electrical relay point known as the AV node (see chapters 1 and 7).

In both roles, digitalis drugs are very useful. But it is estimated that one patient in every five taking digoxin experiences side-effects such as nausea, dizziness and headaches. The concentration at which digoxin starts to poison the body is not much greater than that at which it has beneficial effects. Levels of drug circulating in the body may therefore need to be monitored by blood tests. It is also sometimes recommended that patients take digitalis preparations on certain days of the week only, allowing the body time to excrete the drug.

Drug names in America and other countries

Approved, chemical names of drugs used in America are generally the same as those used in Britain. Where they are not, the similarity is close. For example, frusemide in Britain is known as furosemide in America; and lignocaine as lidocaine.

Many brand names in the two countries are identical. Where they differ, the equivalence of one brand to another can often be seen from the similarity of name. A doctor will usually be able to advise on which section of the book is relevant to a particular medicine.

The availability of drugs differs from one country to another, since methods of approving new products are not the same, and there may be delays in the granting of licences for particular substances to be used. But all of the major types of drug mentioned in this book are found worldwide.

Appendix One

What Happens in Open-heart Surgery?

Together, the lungs and heart do two things: they enrich blood with oxygen (while at the same time removing the waste gas carbon dioxide), and then pump it forcefully around the body. Both functions can now safely and effectively be taken over by a heart–lung machine. Using this technique, called cardiopulmonary bypass, the heart and body are preserved for many hours. Stopping the heart while taking over the patient's circulation by machine is the only way complicated heart surgery can be performed.

Doctors will meet the patient before the day of operation to explain what is to happen. Ideally, people are also shown around the intensive care unit, and encouraged to ask questions and meet patients operated on over the previous few days. This helps reduce the fears and anxiety that patients quite naturally feel.

The procedure itself begins with a sedative drug, given on the ward, to induce calm. The patient is then taken to the operating theatres and met by nurses, technicians and the anaesthetist. The anaesthetist puts the patient to sleep using an intravenous injection, and then inserts fine tubes into the arteries, veins and bladder. These ensure that drugs can be given easily and that the body's vital functions can be monitored and controlled. After this, the patient is washed with sterilising solutions and draped in clean cloths, leaving exposed the area that is to be operated on.

The initial stage of the surgery itself is to enter the chest. A vertical 9-inch (23 cm) cut is made in the skin, and the breastbone is then divided using a fast power saw. The lungs covering the heart are gently moved aside, and the fibrous heart sac revealed. When this is cut through, the surgeon has access to the heart. During these procedures, which take only a few minutes, the heart continues to beat normally. But for the rest of the operation, its work must be taken over by machine.

Blood returning to the heart in the body's major veins enters the right atrium. So that the rest of the heart and lungs can be bypassed, blood is sucked out of this collecting chamber, using one or two large tubes. The blood flows to a machine which enriches it with oxygen, and is then pumped back into the body's system of arteries, usually through a tube placed near the start of the aorta. From there it flows, as it normally would, to the rest of the body.

A tube in the left ventricle of the heart removes any blood that flows into it, and blood seeping into the chest cavity is also sucked up and fed into the circuit of the heart–lung machine. In this way, as little as possible is wasted. Many open-heart operations are performed without need for blood transfusion.

The heart–lung machine ensures that the body and brain are kept well supplied with blood. But what of the heart itself? Several specialised techniques, which have been years in development, are used to protect it. The most common methods involve reducing the oxygen and nutrient demands of the heart by cooling it.

Preserving the heart has several aspects. First, the heart must be stopped suddenly, and not allowed gradually to 'wind down', since any extra beats would use up crucial nutrients in the heart muscle cells and so expose them to damage. This is done using cold solutions (at 4° centigrade) and the chemical element potassium, which brings an abrupt halt to the heart beat. This is called cardioplegia. Secondly, throughout the operation, the heart is kept cool, both by lowering the temperature of the circulating blood and by surrounding the heart with ice-cold fluid. This slows chemical processes within its cells and again limits the damage they suffer.

In most operations using the heart–lung machine, the patient as a whole is also cooled, from the normal 37° centigrade to around 30°. This reduces the body's metabolic rate by around a quarter, and so cuts its demand for oxygen and nutrients. In some very young infants, delicate heart surgery is made easier if the body is further cooled – to around 16°. At this temperature the circulation can be stopped completely without damage to organs such as the brain. In adults, this is not necessary.

Cardiopulmonary bypass keeps the body effectively supplied with oxygenated blood, but the machine is far from a perfect replacement for the heart. Blood is not simply a fluid, but a complex mixture of cells circulating through a system of blood vessels, again composed of living cells, that is finely tuned to the blood's requirements. In particular, blood takes unkindly to contact with the crude artificial metal and plastic surfaces found in tubes and mechanical pumps, and tends to become damaged and form clots. For this reason, drugs that prevent coagulation must be added. Normally, a chemical called heparin is used. At the end of the operation, when we need blood to clot so that the wounds will begin to heal, the effects of heparin must quickly be reversed by the addition of another drug. The substance used is protamine, which is derived from fish.

Procedures such as valve replacement require that the heart itself is opened. The mitral valve, the one that most frequently needs attention, is reached by opening the left atrium. (The aortic valve is operated on from above, through the aorta.) However, the beating chambers are rarely cut into, except for the repair of congenital defects or the structural damage that may occur after a heart attack. Despite the term 'open-heart surgery', bypassing of the coronary arteries does not involve the opening of the heart muscle itself.

The first priority after the main surgery, particularly if the heart has been opened, is to make sure that no air remains inside it. (Air reaching the brain can cause severe damage.) This is done by carefully filling the heart with blood. The heart and the patient are then rewarmed by heating up the blood as it passes through the heart–lung machine.

At this point, the heart may start beating on its own. If it does not, an electric shock is used to jolt it back into action. Once the heart is beating well, it is allowed to take over the circulation. The heart–lung machine is stopped, and its connections to the patient removed. Plastic drainage tubes are placed around the heart and sometimes around the lungs to remove blood that would otherwise accumulate in the first few hours after surgery.

The patient is then 'put back together' again in reverse order: when the surgeon is satisfied the heart is working properly again, the sternum is firmly fastened together with stainless steel wire, and finally the layers of overlying tissue in the chest wall are sutured one by one.

The patient returns asleep to the intensive care unit and spends the first few hours on a ventilator, a 'breathing machine' that rhythmically fills the lungs with air. This involves putting a tube through the mouth and down the windpipe. People on ventilators are not able to talk, but ICU nurses are skilled at communication and can understand patients' complaints and requests. The tube is not uncomfortable, and use of sedative drugs means that most patients have little recollection of events during the 24 hours after surgery.

Patients usually start breathing on their own once they regain consciousness. Where there are no complications, the drips and tubes are removed the next day. Where this might be uncomfortable, pain-killing injections are given beforehand. The patient can then be sent back to a general ward. People who have been very ill before the operation, or whose surgery has been complicated, may need longer on the ventilator and require longer-term support with drugs.

Nowadays, patients are encouraged to be mobile quickly following an operation and are visited early by a physiotherapist who persuades them to breathe deeply and cough, to reduce the chances of chest infection. Most patients can sit out of bed the day following the operation and begin to walk two or three days after surgery. During the first few days, it is important that patients have sufficient pain-killing medication to prevent discomfort, while not having so much that they become drowsy and immobile.

Everyone recovers at their own pace. Some experience little pain, and are quickly active; others take longer. After routine open-heart surgery, most patients are able to go home or to convalescence seven to ten days following their operation. By this stage they will be able to walk freely in the ward, climb at least a flight of stairs, and be well into the first stage of full recovery. Once at home, people are encouraged gradually to increase their activity, under a doctor's guidance, going for regular walks and resuming their normal lifestyle as confidence returns.

The initial impression patients have of the value of their surgery depends on how badly they were affected before the operation. In some patients, particularly those who had severe chest pain, the improvement is immediate and dramatic. Others (including some with valve disease) may have had few symptoms and so notice little difference, yet a condition that would eventually have caused severe problems has been effectively dealt with.

As well as the usual relatively minor discomforts (those that typically occur with heart surgery, especially bypass grafting, are described in chapter 6), some patients develop more serious problems of the kind that may follow any form of major surgery. These tend to happen in people who were particularly sick before their operation, or whose surgery was delayed beyond the point at which it actually became necessary. Possible complications include infections, heart failure, thrombosis (clotting) in the deep veins, kidney failure, disturbances of heart rhythm, jaundice and damage to the brain.

This is a long catalogue, but the most serious complications are uncommon. And though some have lasting effects, they generally delay recovery rather than prevent it. The commonest complication is rhythm disturbance, which occurs in a third of patients following heart surgery. Usually the problem is excessively fast and irregular beating of the atria (atrial fibrillation). This condition responds quickly to drugs and has no long-term effects. A few patients develop excessive bleeding after surgery and have to return to the operating room for it to be dealt with. But this does not usually impair progress.

Elderly patients generally take longer to recover than the young, but the pattern is the same. Many old people have their lives transformed by heart operations, and are once more able to lead an independent existence. Age alone should not be used as an excuse to deny someone access to surgery.

Appendix Two

Inheriting High Cholesterol

Some people inherit the tendency to develop unusually high levels of the various blood fats (or, in medical terms, blood lipids). There are several such conditions, but the one identified by abnormally high cholesterol is by far the most common. As it is passed from one generation to another, the disorder is known as *familial hypercholesterolaemia*. ('Hyper' is a Greek word meaning abnormally increased). There may be as many as 100,000 people with the condition in the UK, roughly one person in 500.

Abnormally high cholesterol levels raise the chances of heart attack, and in men with familial hypercholesterolaemia (or FH) this risk begins to increase appreciably from about the thirtieth year. (In the rest of the male population, a similar risk of heart attack is not reached until the age of 45 or so.) Among women with FH, the risk of serious coronary heart disease increases from about 40 years onwards. Not everyone wth FH will have a heart attack, but the danger is real enough for detection and treatment of the disease to be very worthwhile. Simple blood tests are sufficient to identify the condition.

Early diagnosis means less chance that the disease has already developed in the coronary arteries, and greater opportunity for prevention. People with FH should scrupulously avoid other risk factors for heart disease such as smoking and excess weight.

Diet and cholesterol-lowering drugs

The main aim of treatment is simply to reduce cholesterol levels. Strict adherence to a diet low in saturated (i.e. animal) fat is the usual first step to try. Fresh and frozen fruit and vegetables, cereals and pulses are fine; any dairy products should be low-fat; and white and oily fish, plus fowl, should largely replace red meat.

When diet alone does not control the condition, cholesterol-lowering drugs may be used. These drugs are of two main types: tablets that reduce the amount of cholesterol made by the liver, and powders that increase cholesterol *excretion*. (They are swallowed but not absorbed by the body.)

Examples of tablets are clofibrate (the trade name is Atromid-S) and bezafibrate (Bezalip). Both substances may cause nausea and pain in the abdomen. Clofibrate has the additional problem of sometimes producing gallstones. Using drugs to reduce blood cholesterol seems a simple enough strategy. However, the potential pitfalls are well illustrated by the history of clofibrate. Initial enthusiasm for its use led to a large European trial which published its results in 1978. This showed that men who took clofibrate were less at risk of death from coronary heart disease. However, an unexpectedly large number of the men given the drug died from *other* causes, such that any beneficial effect on the heart was completely negated.

Understandably, this finding switched attention to the alternative form of drug treatment. The powders (really resins) have their effect in the intestine, preventing the absorption of bile, which is then passed in the faeces. Bile is made from cholesterol and its loss causes the body to make more, so using up its cholesterol supplies. Examples are cholestyramine (Questran) and colestipol (Colestid).

Recently, a large American study selected a group of men whose blood cholesterol levels were in the top 5 per cent for the population as a whole, and asked half of them to take a daily dose of cholestyramine. Compared with a control group who received no drug, the men taking cholestyramine had 20 per cent less coronary heart disease. Deaths from heart attack, the incidence of angina and the number of operations to bypass obstructed coronary arteries were all down by the same amount. This is a striking result. However, it is clear that resin preparations are unpalatable to take. Only half the men given cholestyramine in the American study actually took it. And both cholestyramine and colestipol may cause nausea, flatulence, constipation and discomfort in the abdomen. Gradually building up the dose, and mixing the resins well with water may help prevent these adverse effects.

A new generation of drugs is being developed. These will reduce the amount of cholesterol produced by the body, but work in a way which is different from clofibrate. Promising agents are currently under trial.

Screening for FH

The cause of FH lies in an abnormal gene. The result is an excess of low density lipoprotein, which transports cholesterol to the tissues of the body. Where one of these defective genes is inherited, the disease follows the pattern just described. Extremely rarely, a child inherits a defective gene from *both* parents. Heart disease can then become a problem as early as adolescence.

Techniques based on genetic engineering will soon allow such gene defects to be directly identified and traced through the family tree. Until then, we have only indirect methods. If someone has a heart attack in early middle age, there is a possibility that familial hypercholesterolaemia is the cause. It is therefore important to have blood cholesterol levels checked in the rest of the family. There are other signs of the condition. They include the presence of small lumps of deposited fat on the tendons of the hands and heels, and yellow streaks around the eyes. However, these features are not always present, and anyone who thinks they may have the disease should see a doctor.

Appendix Three

Heart Disease and Driving

People should not drive, and should notify the Driver and Vehicle Licensing Centre in Swansea if they:

- have had a heart attack within the past two months;
- have angina frequently while driving;
- are taking drugs that cause vertigo (sensations that the body or the world is spinning), fainting, loss of consciousness, lack of alertness or rapid onset of tiredness;
- have unexplained periods of syncope (temporary loss of consciousness caused by lack of bloodflow to the brain);
- have untreated heartblock (impaired conduction of electrical current through the heart).

Alcohol interacts with many drugs used to treat heart disease, producing further reductions in alertness and slowing reaction time.

Apart from the conditions listed above (based on advice in *Medical Aspects of Fitness to Drive* published by the Medical Commission on Accident Prevention, 1985), it is thought to be generally safe for people with heart disease to drive private vehicles. For example, angina that occurs with strenuous exercise, but not in other circumstances, is not a bar to driving. Most people with disease of the heart valves, or with artificial valves, are able to continue driving (though not, of course, if they experience fits of disabling giddiness or fainting). People with artificial pacemakers are allowed to drive, provided that their underlying heart condition is not dangerous, and that the working of the pacemaker is regularly checked. Driving may be resumed one month after successful implantation of the device. Patients who have had coronary artery surgery may return to driving once they have recovered from the operation.

Regulations are more strict and considerably more complicated when driving involves heavy goods, passenger transport and public service vehicles (including taxis). This is not a complete list, and there are certain exceptions. However, generally speaking, goods and passenger vehicles should not be driven by anyone who has:

- any form of angina;
- evidence on the ECG of lasting damage from a heart attack;
- had more than one heart attack;
- dangerous narrowing of vital sections of the major coronary arteries (revealed by coronary angiography);
- a pacemaker;
- a significantly enlarged heart;
- seriously raised blood pressure.

For people who drive professionally, yearly medical examinations may be necessary to confirm continued fitness to drive.

Professional drivers who have had angioplasty or coronary artery bypass surgery will need to have regular check-ups using angiography and exercise tests to confirm that there is an adequate supply of blood to the heart muscle. As a rough guide, driving may be permitted if yearly checks reveal no symptoms, no ECG signs of inadequate blood supply on exercise testing, no recent heart attack, good pumping performance by the left ventricle and coronary artery grafts that show no signs of becoming blocked by disease.

Appendix Four

Important Dates in the Understanding and Treatment of Heart Disease

1628   William Harvey identifies the function of the heart as the circulation of blood.

1768   Heberden first uses the term 'angina', during his address on chest pain to the London Royal College of Physicians. But it is not realised that coronary artery disease is the cause of angina until the twentieth century.

1770s   Lavoisier and Joseph Priestley discover the role of oxygen.

1785   The medical use of a foxglove extract (digitalis) advocated for heart failure by William Withering.

1816   Invention of the stethoscope in France.

First half of nineteenth century: German physicians Lobstein and Virchow recognise atheroma and thrombosis.

1867   Lauder Brunton (aged 23) working at Edinburgh Royal Infirmary discovers that amyl nitrite relieves angina. It was the first quick and effective therapy. Patients today still use a similar drug, glyceryl trinitrate.

Late 19th century: Development of routine measurement of blood pressure using a sphygmomanometer (Pierre Carl Potain); realisation the heart is worked by electricity; important developments in our understanding (Schiff) of how nerves control the state of the blood vessels.

1892 onwards: Sir James Mackenzie investigates the pulse and rhythms of the heart: the polygraph.

1893 Wilhelm His describes the specialised electrical conduction tissue of the heart.

1900 Willem Einthoven, from Leyden, coins the term electrocardiogram and identifies the contribution of the atria and ventricles to the ECG. His research built upon earlier work by Waller on electrical currents in the heart. It was extended by Sir Thomas Lewis who brought the ECG to the patient's bedside, and identified atrial fibrillation and flutter.

1912 For the first time, a heart attack is diagnosed on the basis of the patient's symptoms, and later confirmed by postmortem examination as being caused by a thrombus blocking a coronary artery. The physician was Herrick, and the place Chicago.

1925 First (closed heart) operation on a narrowed mitral valve.

1929 A German doctor, Forssmann, shows that a fine tube (catheter) inserted into a vein can reach the human heart. This is the basis of many vital diagnostic techniques, including those used to map the coronary arteries, a procedure first performed in 1962.

Second World War: Advances in anaesthesia, antibiotics and blood transfusion lay foundations for safe and widespread cardiac surgery.

1952/3 First successful use of the heart–lung machine to allow prolonged open-heart surgery and first artificial heart valve inserted.

1958 In Sweden, a heart pacemaker is implanted under the skin. The device had to be recharged every week and lasted one year.

1959 First report that a drug (streptokinase) can be used to dissolve clot in blocked coronary arteries. But the technique does not become widely used until the 1980s.

1962 Coronary angiography introduced (see 1929).

1962 Black (working for ICI in Macclesfield) describes the betablockers, a new class of drug that is to become the mainstay of treatment for high blood pressure, and a major help in angina. The discovery by Ahlquist fifteen years earlier of blood vessel receptors paved the way for the development of these drugs.

1966   Radionuclide scanning as a means of diagnosis begins.

1967   Use of a leg vein at the Cleveland Clinic, Ohio, allows surgeons to perform the first coronary artery bypass graft.

1970s Human heart transplantation, started by Christiaan Barnard in South Africa, is developed as a viable surgical procedure.

1977   Angioplasty (widening of a narrowed coronary artery by inflated balloon) performed by Grüntzig.

1981   Simultaneous transplantation of heart and lungs by Reitz and colleagues in Stanford, California. In 1983, the operation is performed for the first time in the UK.

1982   First implantation of an artificial heart, at the University of Utah.

1982   Destruction of part of the conduction system of the heart by massive electric shock (ablation) first used as a treatment for irregular heart rhythm.

Appendix Five

Organisations Involved in Helping People with Heart Disease and in Education and Research

United Kingdom

British Heart Foundation
102 Gloucester Place
London W1H 4DH
Tel.: 01–935 0185

Formed in 1961, the British Heart Foundation finances and encourages research into the causes, diagnosis, prevention and treatment of all forms of heart disease. It also provides cardiac equipment for hospitals and ambulance services in particular need, and publishes a series of advisory pamphlets for the layperson on heart disease and related problems. These are available free of charge from the above address.

Coronary Artery Disease Research Association (CORDA)
47 Wimpole Street
London W1M 7DG
Tel: 01–834 5000

Chest, Heart & Stroke Association
Tavistock House North
Tavistock Square
London WC1H 9JE
Tel.: 01–387 3012

Counselling and many self-help groups throughout the country.

Heartline
Secretary & Co-ordinator of main committee:
Mrs Tricia Pope
12 East Road
Langford
Biggleswade, Beds
Tel.: 0462 700233

An association for the families and friends of children with heart conditions, with many local committees.

The Association for Children with Heart Disorders
National Chairman:
Mrs Rosemary Whitehead
536 Colne Road
Reedsley
Burnley
Tel.: 0282 27500

Zipper Club
Central Committee Chairman:
Mr Doug Carter
9 Foden Avenue
Ipswich, Suffolk
Tel.: 0473 461888

The purpose is to maintain a list of patients who have had cardiac surgery and who would be prepared to meet prospective patients to explain what the operation will entail. There is also a social element. (Several local branches.)

Heart to Heart Group
Secretary:
Mrs J. Richardson
Box No 7
High Street
Pershore, Worcestershire
Tel.: 0905 840446

Counselling service for those about to undergo heart surgery, given by people who have already had similar operations.

Take Heart
Chairman:
Mr George Morland
55 Flaxpiece Road
Claycross
Chesterfield
Tel.: 0246 862462 (evenings)

A club for people who have had a heart attack. Counselling and social activities.

Familial Hypercholesterolaemia Association
Honorary Secretary:
Carolyn Bradbeer
Familial Hypercholesterolaemia Association
PO Box 116
Kidlington
Oxford OX5 1DT
Tel.: 08675 79125

Provide information and support to those found to have FH. Self-help groups on a national basis, keeping in touch with one another through newsletters, regular meetings and the exchange of diet recipes.

Argentina

Argentine Society of Cardiology (Sociedad Argentina de Cardiologia)
Azcuénaga 980/86
1115 Buenos Aires
Tel.: 83 9480

Argentine Heart Foundation (Fundacion Cardiologica Argentina)
Parana 489
Piso 9°
Of. 56
1017 Buenos Aires
Tel.: 46 4221

Australia

The Cardiac Society of Australia and New Zealand
145 Macquarie Street
Sydney
New South Wales 2000
Australia
Tel: 279597

National Heart Foundation of Australia
PO Box 2
Woden
ACT 2606
Australia
Tel.: 82 2144 (Canberra)

Austria

Austrian Heart Foundation (Österreichischer Herzfonds)
Passauer Platz 9
A-1010 Vienna
Tel.: 0222 635550

Belgium

Belgian Heart League (Ligue Cardiologique Belge)
43 rue des Champs Elysees
1050 Brussels
Tel.: 02 6498537

Bangladesh

Bangladesh National Heart Foundation
S Brig (Prof.) Abdul Malik
Director, Institute of Cardiovascular Diseases
Shaheed Suhrawardy Hospital Complex
Sher-e-Rangla Nagar
Dacca 7
Tel.: 311626

Czechoslovakia

Czechoslovak Society of Cardiology
S. Dr J. Fabian
Cardiovascular Research Centre
Institute for Clinical and Experimental Medicine
Videnska 800

Denmark

The Danish Heart Foundation
10 Hauser Plads
DK-1127 Copenhagen K
Denmark
Tel.: 01 131788

Egypt

Egyptian Society of Cardiology
42 Kasr el Eini Street
Dar El-Hekmah
Cairo
Tel.: 23406

France

French Heart Foundation (Fédération de Cardiologie)
50 rue de Rocher
75008 Paris
Tel.: 5225251

Germany

German Society for Circulation Research (Deutsche Gesellschaft für
Herz- und Kreislaufforschung)
Max-Planck-Institut für physiologische und klinische Forschung
W. G. Kerckhoff-Institute

Abt. f. exp. Kardiolog Benekestr. 2
D-6350 Bad Nauheim
Tel.: 06032 345403

Hungary

Hungarian Society of Cardiology
Hungarian Institute of Cardiology
IX Haman Kato ut 29
PO Box 88
Budapest
Tel.: 131 220

India

All India Heart Foundation
4874 Ansari Road
24 Daryaganj
New Delhi 110002
Tel.: 279741

Italy

Italian Society of Cardiology
Corso di Francia 197
00191 Roma
Tel.: 06 3279819

Malaysia

National Heart Association of Malaysia
Physicians Clinic
Hospital Besar
Kuala Lumpur
Tel.: 924180

Netherlands

Netherlands Heart Foundation
Sophialaan 10
2514 JR The Hague
Tel. 070 924292

Dutch Society of Cardiology
Afdeling Cardiologie
Academisch Ziekenhuis
Utrecht
Tel.: 030 372884

Pakistan

Pakistan Heart Foundation
PO Box 244
84 Nishtar Abad
Peshawar
Tel. 72322

Portugal

Portuguese Heart Foundation (Fundacao Portuguesa de Cardiologia)
Terapeutica Medica
Piso 4
University Hospital of Santa Maria
1600 Lisboa
Tel.: 760109 (direct line) 530866 (office) 650686 (home)

Singapore

The Singapore National Heart Association
Colombo Court PO Box 850
Singapore 9117
Tel.: 360644 ext. 280

Spain

Spanish Society of Cardiology (Sociedad Espanola de Cardiologia)
Sagasta 7
Madrid 4
Tel.: 4455726

Switzerland

Swiss Cardiology Foundation
PO Box 176
3000 Bern 15
Tel.: 031 448711

Thailand

The Heart Association of Thailand
Department of Surgery
Faculty of Medicine
Siriraj Hospital
University of Mahidol
Bangkok
Tel.: 282 4141 or 411 1426

Tunisia

Tunisian Society of Cardiology
18 rue de Russie
Tunis
Tel.: 242776

Yugoslavia

Yugoslav Society of Cardiology
Klinika za bolesti srca i reumatizam
Mose Pijade 25
71000 Sarajevo
Tel.: 071 26448

Appendix Six

What to do in an Emergency: Cardio-pulmonary Resuscitation

Someone who has had a heart attack may become unconscious. If the heart has stopped pumping (a condition called cardiac arrest), the person affected will also stop breathing. Their blood is not receiving fresh supplies of oxygen; and it is not being circulated. This situation threatens irreversible damage to the brain. You can help prevent this by artificially inflating the lungs, and by taking over the pumping function of the heart. Since both the heart and the lungs need attention, the techniques together are called *cardio-pulmonary resuscitation*.

The following section shows how to perform cardio-pulmonary resuscitation. First you must take certain common-sense precautions to make sure that it is safe to go to the casualty's aid. Then you must establish that the person you are trying to help really is unconscious. And, finally, you must establish that they are not breathing and/or that the heart has stopped – since a heart attack is only one of many possible causes of unconsciousness. Simple fainting is probably the most frequent, and loss of consciousness during an attack of epilepsy is also common. This step-by-step guide therefore begins with the basics.

Resuscitation for the citizen

Although this information can be used to learn the basic techniques of resuscitation, it must be stated that no instructions, however good, can substitute for a properly administered training course on basic life support techniques. Find out about first-aid courses in your area. Throughout this appendix the casualty is always referred to as male. This is simply for the sake of clarity. In reality the casualty can, of course, be of either sex and of any age. In each case, exactly the same principles apply.

The need for resuscitation

To live we need to have a regular supply of oxygen to all our organs. This is especially important for the brain which will become severely damaged if it is deprived of oxygen for more than a few minutes. To keep the brain supplied with oxygen three things are needed:

A A clear *airway* supplied with oxygen containing air.
B *Breathing* which draws air into the lungs where oxygen can enter the blood stream.
C A *circulation* which requires a pumping heart together with sufficient blood in the blood vessels to carry oxygen from the lungs to the vital organs.

Resuscitation is the term used for the emergency treatment needed to overcome failure of one or all of these functions. It may consist simply of clearing the airway in someone who is choking and placing him in a recovery position, or it may mean the continuing application of artificial breathing and assisted circulation in the casualty. Whatever the circumstances surrounding an unconscious casualty this appendix aims to provide the reader with sufficient knowledge and confidence to resuscitate the casualty should the occasion arise.

Priorities in basic resuscitation

Remember – seconds count.

Approach

Eliminate any danger. Ensure that there is no continuing danger to either yourself or to the casualty from electricity, gas, falling masonry, traffic etc. Establish if the casualty is unconscious by gently shaking him and shouting, 'Are you all right?' Do not aggravate any injuries that he may have, especially in the neck, ribs or limbs, by moving him unnecessarily.

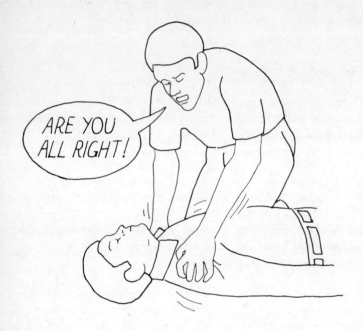

Airway

Once you are certain that the casualty is unconscious you must then check and see whether the airway is clear. Some possible causes of obstruction are:

- The *tongue* may have fallen back blocking the airway in a casualty lying on his back.
- A large chunk of *food* lodged in the throat.
- *Vomit* or *blood* blocking the throat.
- A *foreign body* such as dislodged false teeth.
- Water or weeds collected in the throat from near drowning.

If the casualty is attempting to breathe (look, listen and feel to confirm this) and the airway is clear, turn him on to his side into the *recovery position* and support his chin until help arrives.

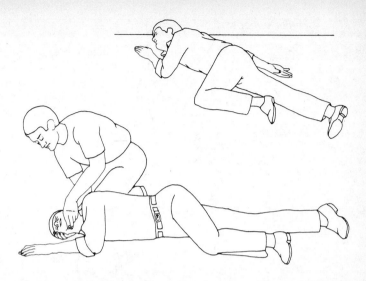

Treatment of an obstructed airway

In an unconscious casualty make sure the airway is open by tilting the head back. This will ensure that the tongue is not obstructing the airway. If the airway remains obstructed after tilting the head back it is possible that vomit, blood or a foreign body is the cause. Remove these by finger sweeps in the mouth if the jaw is relaxed. Try back blows if this is not successful. If the casualty then starts

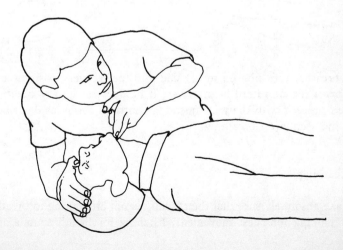

Finger sweeps

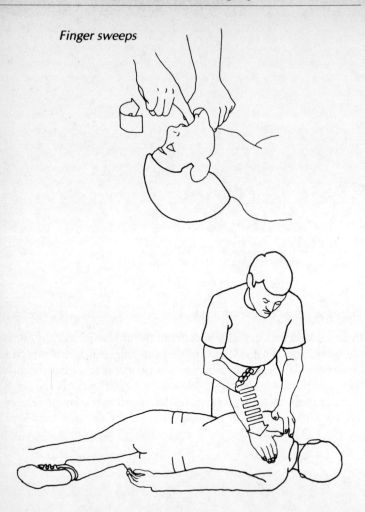

to breathe, turn him on to his side into the recovery position and support his chin until help arrives. If he does *not* start to breathe, then proceed with the recommended course of action as described in the section on breathing.

Breathing

Make absolutely sure that the casualty is not attempting to breathe by looking for chest movement, listening for breath sounds and

Look, listen, feel,

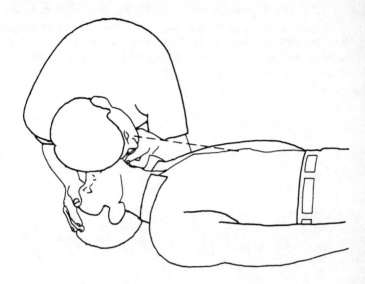

feeling for breath on your cheek. Someone who is not breathing may have a bluish tinge to his lips. There may be several reasons why the casualty has stopped breathing. Some of these are:

- Obstructed airway.
- Stopped heart, e.g., from severe heart attack or electric shock.
- Head injury.
- Chest injury.
- Exposure to poisonous gas (remember to eliminate the danger to yourself first).
- Near drowning.
- Poisoning, e.g., from a drug overdose.

The important thing to remember with all of these causes is that you shouldn't overconcern yourself with the reason why breathing has stopped, only that it has and *you* must act immediately by giving mouth-to-mouth breathing.

Treatment of absent breathing

Expired Air Respiration (known as EAR for short) refers to the breathing given by the rescuer using the mouth-to-mouth method. EAR is performed with the casualty lying on his back, his head tilted back and his mouth open. Kneel by his head and with one hand pinch his nose. With the other support his jaw. Take a breath...

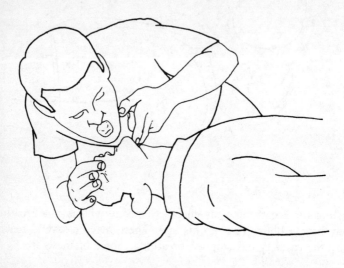

place your mouth completely over the mouth of the casualty making a good seal, and blow. Make sure his chest rises and falls as you perform this operation. Repeat this manoeuvre four times quickly. If the chest does not rise with each breath then either the airway is obstructed or you have not made a good enough seal between your mouth and the casualty's. Try to clear the airway or improve the seal before continuing.

   After doing this check to see if the casualty has started to breathe for himself. If not, check the pulse in the neck (see Circulation). If the casualty is not breathing well, continue mouth-to-mouth breathing at the rate of about 12 breaths per minute in an adult and 20 breaths per minute in infants and small children. If the casualty starts to breathe for himself, turn him on to his side into the recovery position and continue to check that breathing is

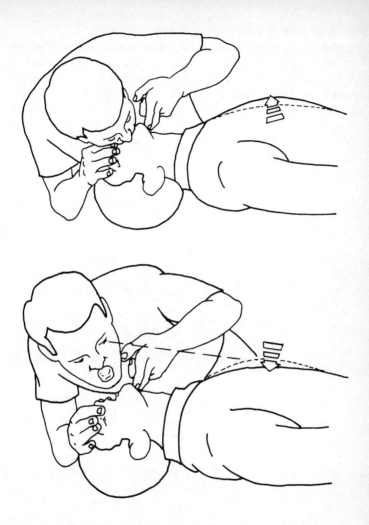

adequate until skilled help arrives. Vomiting often occurs when breathing returns and placing the casualty in the recovery position will prevent him from choking if vomiting does occur.

Circulation

The pulses in the neck are to be found over the carotid arteries which lie on either side of the voice box (Adam's apple) between it and the muscles running up either side of the neck. Feel for your own pulse now to be sure of the precise location. If the casualty has *no pulse*, is *unconscious* and his colour is very *blue*, *grey* or *pale*, then his heart has stopped (cardiac arrest) and an artificial circulation will have to be provided. This is done by external chest compression (known as ECC) which consists of compressing the chest rhythmically to squeeze blood out of the heart and into the circulation.

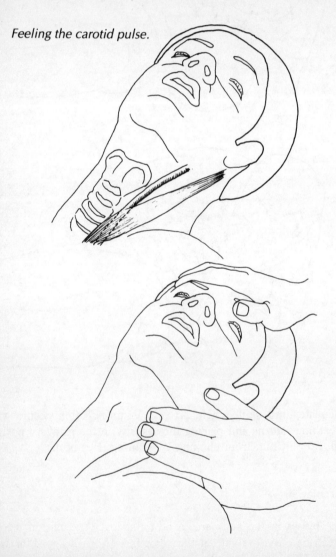

Feeling the carotid pulse.

In all cases where the heart has stopped, breathing will also stop within a minute so these casualties will need both expired air respiration and external chest compression. This combination is known as Cardio-Pulmonary Resuscitation (or CPR for short). Some causes of cardiac arrest are:

- Heart attack.
- Severe blood loss.
- Severe head injury.
- Near drowning.
- Overdose of poison or noxious gas (remember to eliminate any dangers to yourself first).
- Electric shock (eliminate danger – switch off or move the casualty away from the source).

As with breathing the important thing to remember with all of these causes is not to overconcern yourself with them. The casualty's heart has stopped and *you* must therefore act immediately by giving CPR (i.e., mouth-to-mouth respiration *and* external chest compression performed together). Any serious bleeding that the casualty may have must be stopped immediately otherwise there will not be enough blood in the circulation to carry oxygen. (See 'Bleeding').

Treatment of cardiac arrest

External chest compression is performed with the patient lying on his back and on a firm surface. By rhythmically pressing the breast bone towards the backbone, the heart is compressed and made to pump blood.

ECC

Kneeling by the side of the casualty locate the base of the breast bone. Place one hand two fingers breadth above this point – over the lower third of the breast bone – in the midline (see p. 206). Place your other hand on top of the first and with your elbows straight bring your shoulders up until they are directly over the casualty's chest. Rhythmically depress and release the breast bone four to five centimetres (one to two inches). Proportionally less movement is needed for children and babies. Remember that both mouth-to-mouth respiration and external chest compression are

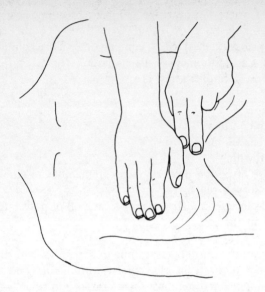

needed in a cardiac arrest. The exact technique will depend on whether you are on your own or if there is another rescuer to help. If you are on your own, alternate 15 compressions (at the rate of about 80 per minute) with two breaths. If there are two rescuers present one should carry out external chest compression uninterrupted at a rate of about 60 per minute whilst the other should provide one breath every fifth compression. The rescuer performing the compressions should not pause at any time for the rescuer performing mouth-to-mouth respiration.

The rescuer performing mouth-to-mouth respiration should check every minute or two for the return of pulse, breathing and colour. If the pulse and breathing return, turn the casualty into the recovery position but continue to *observe him carefully* until skilled help arrives. In young children and babies the breaths used in mouth-to-mouth respiration should be proportionately less. External chest compressions in children are performed with one hand at the rate of 80 or 90 per minute and in infants with the fingertips at the rate of 100 per minute (see p. 209). In babies the rescuer performing mouth-to-mouth respiration should place his mouth over the mouth *and* nose of the baby.

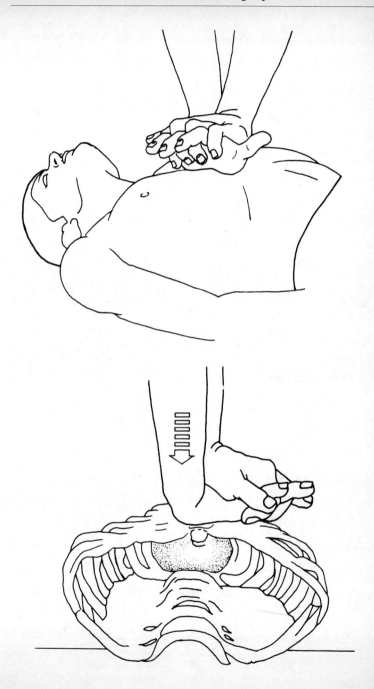

15 compressions to two breaths.

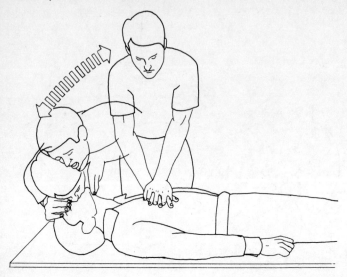

Five compressions to one breath.

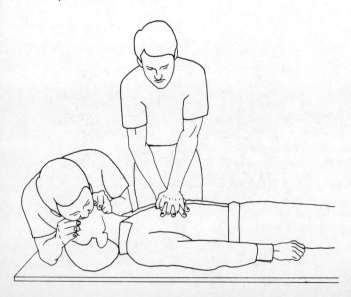

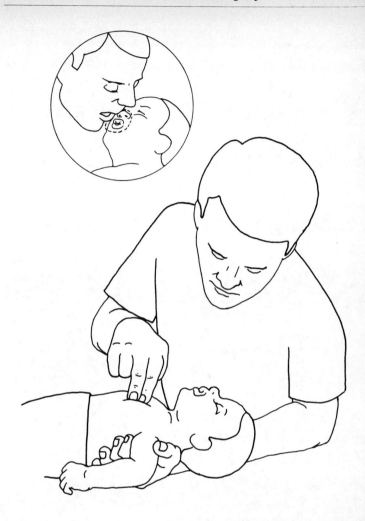

Bleeding

In casualties where the cardiac arrest is associated with blood loss it is necessary to control any obvious heavy bleeding by direct pressure over the wound. Use a pad or a dressing if available. If at all possible, the wound should be elevated to a position which allows gravity to act against the blood flow. The legs of the casualty should also be raised to allow the blood to drain from them to the vital organs.

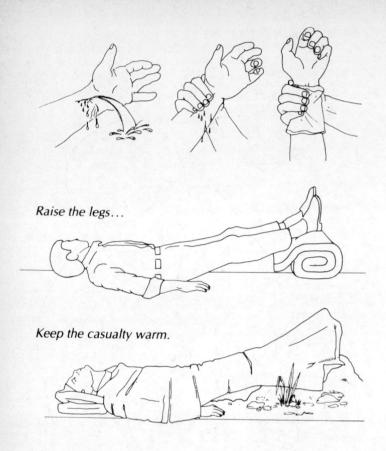

Raise the legs...

Keep the casualty warm.

Summary of resuscitation procedure

1 Remember – seconds count.
2 Eliminate danger.
3 Establish unconsciousness – shake and shout.
4 Clear the airway – tilt the head back, remove foreign material and support the chin. Check for breathing.
5 If breathing, turn the casualty into the recovery position.
6 If not breathing, give mouth-to-mouth respiration.
7 Check for a pulse in the neck.

8 If no pulse, begin external compression together with mouth-to-mouth respiration (C.P.R.)
- One rescuer – 15 compressions to 2 breaths.
- Two rescuers – 5 compressions to 1 breath.
9 Stop obvious heavy bleeding.
10 Continue until either:
- Pulse and breathing are restored.
- A doctor or qualified help assumes responsibility for the casualty.
- You are completely exhausted and unable to continue.

These instructions are reproduced by kind permission of the Resuscitation Council (UK). Copies of the booklet *Resuscitation for the Citizen* are available from the Resuscitation Council, Department of Anaesthetics, Royal Postgraduate Medical School, Hammersmith Hospital, London W12 0HS. Original diagrams courtesy of A. S. Laerdal, Stavanger, Norway.

Glossary of Major Medical Terms

ambulatory (24-hour) monitoring   Recording the heart's electrical activity over long periods with a portable ECG device.

aneurysm   A weak point in an artery or heart wall which 'balloons out' and may burst.

angina   Chest pain or ache (usually brought on by exercise or emotion and usually relieved by rest) showing that heart muscle is receiving insufficient oxygen.

angiography   Aid to diagnosis in which the blood vessels (especially the coronary arteries) are revealed by injection of fluid that shows up on X-rays.

angioplasty   Process of dilating blood vessels (especially the coronary arteries) by inflation of a small balloon catheter.

aorta   The single, large artery starting at the left ventricle. From the aorta, blood is distributed to the body.

arrest   Stopping of the heart.

arrhythmia   Abnormal rhythm of the heart.

artery   Vessel taking blood from the heart.

atheroma   Mixture of fat and blood components deposited along the walls of arteries.

atherosclerosis   Narrowing of the arteries by atheroma.

atrium (atria)   The chambers of the heart that collect blood.

bradycardia   Abnormally slow heart rate.

Bruce protocol   A form of exercise test (*see* Exercise test).

calcification   Hardening due to deposits of calcium.

cardiac   Relating to the heart.

cardiac massage   Rhythmic pressure on the chest that may restart a heart that has stopped beating.

cardiovascular Relating to the heart and blood vessels.

cardioversion Delivery of an electric shock to stop abnormal heart rhythm.

catecholamines The hormones adrenaline and noradrenaline that increase the activity of the heart and prepare the body for fight or flight.

catheter A fine tube inserted into the body. Cardiac catheterisation is the process of introducing a catheter into the blood vessels and the heart, usually to help assess the heart's function or the condition of the coronary arteries.

cerebrovascular Relating to the brain's blood supply. Cerebrovascular accident is a medical term for stroke.

chordae Tendons connecting the flaps of valves to the heart wall.

congenital Present at birth.

coronary arteries Blood vessels supplying the heart muscle.

coronary artery bypass graft (CABG) An operation to bypass obstructions in narrowed coronary arteries.

coronary thrombosis Formation of a clot (thrombus) that blocks flow of blood through a coronary artery and so leads to death of heart muscle (myocardial infarction).

diastole The period in the heart cycle when heart muscle is relaxed and the ventricles fill with blood. Blood pressure is lowest at this point.

defibrillation Delivery of a strong electric shock to the heart to stop a life-threatening abnormality of heart rhythm.

dysrhythmia Abnormal rhythm of the heart.

ECG or EKG Electrocardiogram: record of the electrical activity that drives the heart.

echocardiography Aid to diagnosis in which images of the heart are obtained using sound waves.

electrode Contact (usually metal) used to record electrical activity (as in the ECG) or deliver electric current (as in a pacemaker).

embolism Sudden blockage of an artery by a clot, bacteria or bubble of air borne on the stream of blood.

exercise test ECG record of the electrical activity of the heart during gradually increasing exercise.

fibrillation Abnormally fast, uncoordinated beating of a heart chamber. Fibrillation of the ventricles quickly leads to death unless the condition can be reversed.

fibrosis Formation of scar-like tissue consisting mostly of fibres.

fluoroscope An X-Ray device used when catheters or pacemaker wires are being positioned in the heart.

haemoglobin Protein pigment in red blood cells that carries oxygen and carbon dioxide.

heart block When the normal electrical impulses that drive the heart fail to pass from the atria to the ventricles.

heart failure Inability of the heart to pump sufficient blood to meet the demands of the circulation. The cause may be problems of the heart muscle, valves or electrical system.

heart–lung machine Mechanical device used to take over the pumping function of the heart and the oxygenating function of the lungs.

Holter monitoring Recording the ECG over long periods with a portable device while the patient moves about.

hyper- Term suggesting 'too much', as in *hypertension* meaning abnormally high blood pressure, and *hyperlipidaemia*, high levels of fats circulating in the blood; and *hypertrophy*, abnormal enlargement.

hypo- Term suggesting 'too little', as in *hypotension*, i.e. abnormally low blood pressure.

incompetence (of a heart valve) Leakage.

infarction Death of tissue from lack of oxygen following interruption to its blood supply.

ischaemia Lack of blood supply (usually leading to damage if prolonged).

ischaemic heart disease Narrowing of the coronary arteries restricting blood flow and so oxygen supply; the condition leading to angina and heart attack.

IV Intravenous; into a vein.

lipids Fats

myocardium Heart muscle.

myocardial infarction Death of heart muscle following interruption to its blood supply.

occlusion Blockage.

oedema Abnormal accumulation of fluid, usually in lungs (pulmonary oedema) or around ankles, and a symptom of heart failure (and many other conditions).

pacemaker Electrical device used to regulate the heart rate, and usually implanted under the patient's skin.

plaque Accumulation of deposits (usually of fat and blood products) along the artery wall).

prognosis The future course of the illness. A favourable prognosis offers good chance of recovery.

prophylaxis Prevention.

pulmonary Relating to the lungs.

pulmonary artery Blood vessel leading from the right ventricle to the lungs.

pulmonary embolism Sudden blockage of the pulmonary artery or its branches by a clot, air bubble etc. borne on the stream of blood.

pulmonary veins Blood vessels leading from the lungs to the left atrium.

regurgitation Leakage of blood through heart valves.

septum Muscle wall dividing the left from the right side of the heart.

sinus node Collection of cells in the right atrium whose regular electrical discharges set the rhythm for the healthy heart.

stenosis Abnormal narrowing (especially of the passage through a heart valve).

stress test ECG record of the electrical activity of the heart during gradually increasing exercise.

stroke Loss of movement or sensation following damage to an area of the brain caused by the blockage or bursting of one of its blood vessels.

syncope Temporary loss of consciousness caused by insufficient blood flow to the brain, often due to an abnormality of heart rhythm.

systole The period in the heart cycle when the ventricles contract to expel blood. Blood pressure is at its peak during this phase.

tachycardia Abnormally fast heart rate.

thrombosis Formation of a clot (thrombus) that often leads to blockage of a blood vessel.

thrombolysis Dissolving a blood clot.

triglycerides Fatty substances in the blood. Abnormally high levels may contribute to the formation of atheroma and gradual obstruction of arteries.

treadmill test Record of the electrical activity of the heart during gradually increasing exercise.

ultrasound Aid to diagnosis in which images of the internal organs (including the heart) are obtained using sound waves.

veins Vessels that return blood to the heart.

ventricle(s) The main beating chambers of the heart.

ventriculogram Image used in diagnosis showing the shape and size (and hence also the performance) of the ventricles.

Index